100 Questions & Answers About Biliary Cancer

Ghassan K. Abou-Alfa, MD

Associate Attending
GI Medical Oncology Service
Memorial Sloan-Kettering Cancer Center
Associate Professor of Medicine
Weill Medical College of Cornell University
New York, NY

Eileen M. O'Reilly, MD

Associate Attending
GI Medical Oncology Service
Memorial Sloan-Kettering Cancer Center
Associate Professor of Medicine
Weill Medical College of Cornell University
New York, NY

JONES & BARTLETT
L E A R N I N G

World Headquarters
Jones & Bartlett Learning
5 Wall Street
Burlington, MA 01803
978-443-5000
info@jblearning.com
www.jblearning.com

Jones & Bartlett Learning books and products are available through most bookstores and online booksellers. To contact Jones & Bartlett Learning directly, call 800-832-0034, fax 978-443-8000, or visit our website, www.jblearning.com.

Production Credits

Executive Acquisitions Editor: Nancy Anastasi Duffy
Production Assistant: Alex Schab
Manufacturing and Inventory Control Supervisor: Amy Bacus
Composition: Jason Miranda, Spoke & Wheel
Cover Design: Stephanie Torta

Photo Research and Permissions Coordinator: Lauren Miller
Cover Image: Top courtesy of Marianne Clement; Bottom courtesy of Rick Pollock
Printing and Binding: Edwards Brothers Malloy
Cover Printing: Edwards Brothers Malloy

ISBN: 978-1-284-02537-8

6048

Printed in the United States of America
17 16 15 14 13   10 9 8 7 6 5 4 3 2 1

CONTENTS

In October of 2005 our family gathered together at our brother's request. Mark and his wife, Marianne, expecting their fourth child in a few weeks, told us that he had been diagnosed with inoperable and incurable bile duct cancer, called Cholangiocarcinoma.

That evening, I got on the computer and began what would become a 15 month journey of intense research, networking, and soul-searching. Our family got organized and made a plan. Mark would look after his personal mental and physical well-being; Marianne would take care of their newborn son, Lucas, and their other three children: Patrick, Chase, and Tessa. Our mother, father, two sisters and I would divide and conquer everything else.

The first weeks and months of research were difficult as we realized there simply wasn't much information to be found, or it was buried in PubMed. Bit by bit, information was cobbled together from the dozens of conversations we had with physicians across the country who were willing to take a look at Mark's medical records. Pieces of information and additional research from other patients were assessed and integrated where applicable.

We worked long hours trying to discover hope for Mark, his family, and ourselves. In the end, our family did not receive what it had hoped and worked for, but we did receive comfort in answers to prayer, clear direction from above, and abundant love and support from the many patients, friends, and physicians we had connected with in the process.

As heart-wrenching as this journey was for us, Mark was determined that no one else should have to invest the time and effort we did to gather information and surround themselves with an empathetic community. Somehow, he wanted us to find a way to endow others with the hope and support he had experienced.

This book, authored by Dr. Abou-Alfa and Dr. O'Reilly and supported by The Cholangiocarcinoma Foundation, will be a valuable resource in the hands of patients and caregivers. It will streamline information gathering, which in the past was an exhausting and overwhelming part of being diagnosed with any of the biliary cancers, including intrahepatic and extrahepatic cholangiocarcinoma, and gallbladder cancer. We are so pleased with the result and grateful to have the opportunity to present this book to you.

Stacie Clements Lindsey
President & Founder,
The Cholangiocarcinoma Foundation

It was just after Thanksgiving, in the Fall of 2008, that I was diagnosed with cholangiocarcinoma. Fortunately, I live in the New York metropolitan area and was able to go to Memorial Sloan-Kettering Cancer Center. They installed a stent in my bile duct to allow the bile to flow. I met with my new oncologist, Dr. Abou-Alfa, and we discussed the combination of drugs that he proposed using as the best option for my condition. The treatments were effective, causing the tumor to shrink and it continues to remain stable in size. Having lived with this condition for the past several years, Dr. Abou-Alfa thought it might be helpful for me to share some of my experiences and thoughts around biliary cancer. You will find my comments on many of the areas addressed in this book. I hope they will be of value for you and will encourage you to fight the battle.

Gary Rosen

PART ONE

The Basics

What is bile and what are bile ducts?

What does the gallbladder do?

What are biliary cancers?

More...

1. What is cancer?

Cancer

The growth and division of cells in an unregulated fashion, which impedes the normal cell cycle.

Cell cycle

The control of cells by orderly signals that indicate when they should grow and divide.

Metastasis

The process of cancer cells invading other organs directly or spreading via the blood stream and lymphatic channels to other areas of the body.

Gallbladder cancer

Cancer that starts in the gallbladder.

Cancer is the growth and division of cells in an unregulated fashion. Normally, orderly signals control cells and indicate when they should grow and divide. We call this natural turnover the **cell cycle**. Normal cells are usually in a resting phase of the cell cycle—performing their usual functions. They grow and divide only when natural chemical "messengers" in the body tell them to do so, and they stop growing and die when internal regulatory mechanisms call for it.

Cells become cancerous when the regulatory mechanisms that control cell growth don't work, such as when the normal control points in the cell cycle are turned off or restrained. They continue to grow uncontrollably and often in a disorganized fashion, eventually forming a malignant tumor, or mass of cancerous cells, within an organ. These cells can interrupt the normal function of the organ or system in which they form by crowding out normal cells or blocking passageways from one organ to another (e.g., when a tumor of the digestive tract blocks food from passing through the intestine).

Unlike normal cells, cancer cells also have the ability to invade other organs directly or to spread via the blood stream and lymphatic channels to other areas of the body, a process called **metastasis** (see Question 19).

The origin of the cancer refers to the primary site of origin of the cancer (thus, **gallbladder cancer** starts off in the gallbladder). Secondary sites, or metastases, are the places where the cancer has spread. A cancer is always referred to by the primary site of origin, regardless of the site of spread (e.g., cholangiocarcinoma spread to the lung is called metastatic cholangiocarcinoma and not lung cancer). Knowing the original location of the cancer is important because different cancers respond to different treatments; for example, a drug that works well on lung cancer may not work on gallbladder cancer that has spread to the lung.

2. What is bile and what are bile ducts?

Bile is a liquid secreted by the liver that helps you digest food, especially fatty foods. Bile is carried through very fine tubes throughout the liver called **bile ducts**. Bile ducts join together like a branching tree into larger ducts until they exit the liver through a main duct called the **common hepatic duct**. The common hepatic duct joins another duct called the **cystic duct**, which leads from the gallbladder, where bile is stored. The common hepatic duct and cystic duct join together to form the **common bile duct**, which opens into a specific segment of the intestine leading from the stomach called the **duodenum**. Before reaching the duodenum, the common bile duct travels for a short time inside the pancreas (another vital organ that helps digest food and control blood sugar in your body). Bile is produced on demand every time you eat, especially after you eat fatty food. This collection of bile ducts is called the **biliary tree** (See **Figure 1**).

THE BASICS

Bile
A liquid secreted by the liver that helps in the digestion of food, particularly fatty foods.

Bile ducts
Thin tubes in the liver that carry bile.

Common hepatic duct
The main duct of the liver through which bile ducts exit.

Cystic duct
A duct that leads from the gallbladder and joins with the common hepatic duct.

Common bile duct
A duct that is formed by the joining of the common hepatic duct and the cystic duct. The common bile duct travels through the pancreas and opens into the duodenum.

Duodenum
The first section of the small intestine.

Biliary tree
The collection of all the bile ducts.

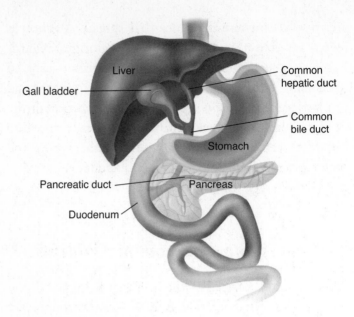

Figure 1 Biliary Tree

3. What does the gallbladder do?

The **gallbladder** is a small, round, and hollow organ that stores bile and sits outside the liver in the upper right side of the abdomen. The gallbladder squirts bile into a section of the intestine (duodenum) after eating, with more being squirted after eating fatty food. Stones can form in the gallbladder, which can block the drainage of bile from the gallbladder, resulting in pain, fever, inflammation of the pancreas, and a condition called jaundice (see Question 84). Jaundice can cause the skin and eyes to appear yellow and urine to become dark or tea-colored. In these latter situations, the gallbladder is removed by a small **laparoscopic** (keyhole) surgery. A person can live a normal life without a gallbladder.

4. Are there different types of biliary cancers?

There are three main types of bile duct cancers that are named based on their site of origin in the biliary tree. Cancer that arises from the major bile ducts inside the liver is called an **intrahepatic cholangiocarcinoma**. If the cancer begins at the bile ducts outside the liver it is referred to as **extrahepatic bile duct cancer**. These extrahepatic bile duct cancers are located at the confluence of the liver and the extrahepatic bile ducts. Extrahepatic choangiocarcinoma is further subdivided as either peripheral or hilar; the later also called **Klatskin tumors**. Cancer originating at the gallbladder is called gallbladder cancer. Gallbladder cancers, like the other types of bile duct cancers, are classified as **adenocarcinomas**, or glandular cancers.

Additionally, there are some rare types of gallbladder cancers, such as squamous cell carcinoma and neuroendocrine carcinoma, as well as a mixture of the two. Your doctor will direct therapy based on the type of gallbladder cancer you have.

The differentiation between the three most common types of **biliary cancers** is in part location based, and this is reflected by the different types of surgeries used to manage each. These surgeries will be discussed further in Part 5. At the present, the treatments used when biliary cancers are not operable are similar. However, there has been evidence that these three types of bile duct cancer differ at a genetic level and may require different types of therapy in the future.

THE BASICS

Intrahepatic cholangio-carcinoma

Cancer that arises from the major bile ducts inside the liver.

Extrahepatic bile duct cancer

Cancer that involves the bile ducts outside the liver. These cancers are found at the joining of the liver and the extrahepatic bile ducts and are also known as Klatskin tumors.

Klatskin tumor

Extrahepatic bile duct cancers that are located very close to where the bile ducts exit the liver.

Adenocarcinoma

Type of cancer that develops in organs that have a tube structure, like the colon, or bile ducts. It is also called glandular cancer.

Biliary cancer

Cancer of the bile ducts.

PART TWO

Risk Factors

How common is cholangiocarcinoma
and what are the risks for developing it?

How common is extrahepatic bile duct cancer
and what are the risks for developing it?

How common is gallbladder cancer
and what are the risks for developing it?

More...

Cholangio-carcinoma

Cancer that originates in the major bile ducts in the liver.

Primary sclerosing cholangitis

A condition in which bile ducts become inflamed and blocked that can eventually lead to cholangiocarcinoma.

Choledochal cysts

A condition in which bile ducts dilate and make cyst-like structures; can be a risk factor for cholangiocarcinoma. Also known as Caroli disease.

Caroli disease

A condition, also known as choledochal cysts, in which bile ducts dilate and make cyst-like structures; can be a risk factor for cholangiocarcinoma.

Ulcerative colitis

A condition in which the gut or intestines is/are inflamed; can be a risk factor for cholangiocarcinoma.

5. How common is cholangiocarcinoma and what are the risks for developing it?

Cholangiocarcinoma is more common in men than women and generally occur in patients between the ages of 50 and 70. Risk factors are mainly certain inflammatory conditions that can affect the bile ducts in the liver. These conditions include **primary sclerosing cholangitis**, a condition in which the bile ducts may become inflamed and subsequently blocked, and **choledochal cysts**, also called **Caroli disease**, which causes bile ducts to dilate and form cyst-like structures. An inflammation of the gut, or intestines, called **ulcerative colitis**, which is related to a process called **sclerosing cholangitis**, can also be a risk factor for developing cholangiocarcinoma.

Infections, particularly in Asia, may also be responsible for the development of cholangiocarcinoma. These include bile duct infections, which are often caused by a worm commonly found in Thailand and other parts of Asia, typhoid fever, hepatitis B, and hepatitis C.

Chemicals including nitrosamines, dioxin, asbestos, and polychlorinated biphenyls may also cause cholangiocarcinoma. Cigarette smoking has been implicated as well.

6. Can cholangiocarcinoma occur along with primary liver cancer or hepatocellular carcinoma?

Close to one in six patients who have primary liver cancer, also called **hepatocellular carcinoma**, may develop cholangiocarcinoma as well. Obviously, having the two cancers side by side creates certain challenges regarding management and treatment. Of particular concern is the associated **cirrhosis** or liver failure that commonly accompanies primary liver cancer. Based on how much of an underlying liver reserve the body has, cirrhosis can severely limit or guide treatment options.

7. How common is extrahepatic bile duct cancer and what are the risks of developing it?

Extrahepatic bile duct cancer is not as common as intrahepatic bile duct cancer. As it is less common, its risk factors are not understood as well, though the inflammatory conditions mentioned in Question 5 typically apply. Extrahepatic biliary cancers typically come to medical attention after the development of jaundice due to blockage of the duct by the tumor. By contrast, intrahepatic bile duct cancers do not usually cause jaundice because they do not block the outer ducts.

8. How common is gallbladder cancer and what are the risks of developing it?

Gallbladder cancer is 3–6 times more common in women than in men, and the risk of developing it increases with age. South America and India have the highest incidence of gallbladder cancer in women worldwide. A high incidence is also noted among Native Americans and Mexican Americans in the United States. The causes behind the increased risk of developing gallbladder cancer among women and in certain regions of the world appear to be related to the increased risk of developing gallstones and inflammation of the gallbladder among those populations.

RISK FACTORS

Sclerosing cholangitis
A condition in which bile ducts narrow, causing irregularities.

Hepatocellular carcinoma
Cancer that starts in the liver.

Cirrhosis
A liver disease, often a result of alcoholism or hepatitis that can complicate the treatment of biliary cancers.

The causes behind the increased risk of developing gallbladder cancer among women and in certain regions of the world appear to be related to the increased risk of developing gallstones and inflammation of the gallbladder among those populations.

Porcelain gallbladder

Calcification in the wall of the gallbladder.

Obesity can lead to gallbladder cancer.

Another risk factor is a condition called **porcelain gallbladder**, in which the gallbladder wall is calcified. Similar conditions to those associated with cholangiocarcinoma and extrahepatic bile duct cancer, like choledochal cysts or Caroli disease, in addition to other anatomical variations that can lead to inflammation, can cause gallbladder carcinoma. Obesity is also associated with gallbladder cancer.

9. Should I go for genetic testing?

Genetic testing

Direct examination of a person's DNA obtained from blood, the mouth, or a tumor. Genetic testing is valuable when concerning heritable diseases and certain cancers.

Biliary cancers have not yet benefited from genetic testing, as it remains unclear what should be looked for.

Mutation

Change.

Genetic testing is a sophisticated process that involves direct examination of genetic material, or DNA, which is obtained from the blood, a tumor, or the lining of the mouth. Genetic testing has proven valuable in detecting the risk of certain genetically inherited diseases and cancers. Biliary cancers have not yet benefited from genetic testing, as it remains unclear what should be looked for. Nonetheless, in certain situations, your doctor may recommend genetic testing because of the possible association of your cancer with other specific conditions or because you may have a strong family history of cancer. For example, people of Eastern European Ashkenazi heritage and with a family or personal history of breast, ovarian, pancreatic, prostate, or other cancers may harbor a BRCA gene **mutation** (change). The BRCA 1 and 2 gene changes can increase the risk of developing biliary cancers, although the overall contribution of the changes in the BRCA genes to the occurrence of biliary cancers is very small.

Gary Rosen's comment:

During my initial discussions at Memorial Sloan-Kettering Cancer Center (MSKCC), I brought up the fact that my mother, father, brother, aunt, and uncle all had different forms of cancer. As I am of Ashkenazi descent, it was suggested that I might want to go for genetic testing. The result was both enlightening and frightening. It was determined that I am BRCA 2 positive. The enlightening was that it gave some insight as to my family history and offered a potential alternative treatment. The frightening was that I have two daughters and I was terrified that I might have passed this on to them. Ironically, both of my daughters (in their 30s) found this to be a relief because they had grown up with a dark cloud over their heads, assuming cancer in their future. The good new is they were tested and both came up negative.

10. Does my family need to be screened for biliary cancers?

Relatively little is known about the genetic inheritance of biliary cancers or even about predisposed conditions that may lead to biliary cancers (see Question 9). In addition, both the risk factors that may lead to the development of biliary cancers, genetic or otherwise, are poorly understood.

As a result, patients can discover that they have an advanced stage of this cancer without having shown any symptoms. It is therefore very difficult to recommend any screening methods for biliary cancers. Even in areas with a high presence of gallbladder cancer and in patients who are considered high risk (for which a doctor may recommend regular ultrasound screenings), there is no proof of any effective screening programs at the present.

11. Should my family members have their gallbladders removed if I have gallbladder cancer?

Because of the strong association of gallbladder cancer with gallstone disease, one might think that removing the gallbladder in patients with gallstones may reduce the risk of gallbladder cancer. Unfortunately, this has not been proven to be correct, and thus, preventive removal of the gallbladder based on risk of developing gallbladder cancer is not a standard practice. The only exception is when there is calcification seen in the wall of the gallbladder (porcelain gallbladder), in which case, preventive removal of the gallbladder removal is justified. However, a family history of gallbladder cancer or any other bile duct cancer does not justify the removal of the gallbladder or the bile ducts in other members of the family.

PART THREE

Diagnosis and Staging

What are the signs and symptoms of cholangiocarcinoma?

How is cholangiocarcinoma diagnosed?

What are the symptoms of extrahepatic bile duct cancer?

More...

Jaundice

A condition marked by a yellowing of the skin and eyes and a darkening of the urine, possibly due to an obstruction of the bile ducts.

Ascites

A condition in which the abdomen is distended with fluid.

Ultrasound

A medical imaging test that produces images of the internal organs.

Computed tomography (CT) scan

An X-ray that produces images of sections of the body.

Magnetic resonance imaging (MRI)

A medical imaging test that produces images of the internal organs.

Unknown primary

A cancer for which the origin is unknown.

Whole body CT scan

An X-ray that produces images of larger portions of the body than a regular CT scan, covering the chest, abdomen, and pelvis.

12. What are the signs and symptoms of cholangiocarcinoma?

When a cholangiocarcinoma tumor forms in the bile ducts within the liver, it is called intrahepatic cholangiocarcinoma. Most intrahepatic and some extrahepatic cholangiocarcinomas present with no symptoms and can be found incidentally when imaging is performed for some other reason. Sometimes the liver blood tests will be elevated without jaundice, which can lead your doctor to investigate. However, when symptoms are present, they may include abdominal pain and/or **jaundice**. Also, during a physical examination, your doctor may notice that your liver is enlarged, or that your abdomen is distended with fluid, a condition called **ascites** (see Question 88).

13. How is cholangiocarcinoma diagnosed?

Cholangiocarcinoma is commonly found incidentally or by chance, such as finding a liver mass while undergoing an **ultrasound**, a **computed tomography (CT) scan**, or a **magnetic resonance imaging (MRI)** for other symptoms or medical problems. You may hear the term **unknown primary**, which means cancer is present but of an unknown point of origin. As many cancers can spread or metastasize to the liver and look like a cholangiocarcinoma, it is common for your doctor to perform extra tests to check if there is another site of origin (where the cancer started) of the cancer within your body. Such tests may include a **whole body CT scan** that covers the chest, abdomen, and pelvis. You may also have a **colonoscopy** and/or an **esophagogastroduodenoscopy (EGD)** to look at the inside of your intestinal tract. Occasionally, a **positron emission tomography (PET) scan** will be performed. A PET scan involves injecting a sugar tracer into the body, causing cancer cells to light up and possibly indicate where the cancer may be coming from. However, inflammatory conditions can mimic a cancer on a PET scan, so these scans require careful interpretation. Women and sometimes men may undergo mammograms as well. If no other primary tumor site is found, then it may be decided that the primary site, or site of origin, is within the bile ducts (cholangiocarcinoma).

Gary Rosen's comment:

In the fall of 2008, I noticed that my urine was getting quite dark and I was itching all over my body. As time progressed, I also became quite jaundiced. I went to my general practitioner, who took a blood test. The readings on my liver were somewhat alarming to him, so he scheduled me for an ultrasound. They saw a mass in the upper middle part of my liver. I next went for an MRI. When he saw the results, his words of advice were: "This doesn't look good and shouldn't be handled locally." We contacted MSKCC and went in for a consultation. Over the next few weeks, they performed a CT scan and biopsy and inserted a stent in my bile duct. The itching lessened and my urine began to look more normal, and my jaundiced condition went away.

14. What are the symptoms of extrahepatic bile duct cancer?

While intrahepatic cholangiocarcinoma does not usually cause jaundice-like symptoms, if you have extrahepatic bile duct cancer, it is more likely that your symptoms are most likely related to the obstruction of the bile ducts because of the cancer. You may become jaundiced and

Colonoscopy

Endoscopic examination of the bowl with a camera on a flexible tube passed through the anus. It can be used for visual diagnosis and biopsies.

Esophagogastro-duodenoscopy (EGD)

A minimally invasive diagnostic endoscopic procedure that visualizes the upper part of the gastrointestinal tract up to the duodenum.

Positron emission tomography (PET) scan

A test that involves the injection of a sugar tracer into the body, which causes cancer cells to light up, in hopes of identifying the origin of the cancer.

DIAGNOSIS AND STAGING

may experience itching. You may have right upper side abdominal pain, experience lost appetite and weight loss, or feel generally unwell. To relieve the jaundice, you may require a **endoscopic retrograde cholangiopancreatography (ERCP)** or a percutaneous intervention. In both procedures, a **stent** or metal tube is inserted into the bile duct in order to open it, allowing bile to flow and relieve the jaundice. As with any procedure or surgery, when a procedure of this kind is performed, bacteria may be introduced to the normally sterile bile duct system. This can sometimes lead to infection. Your doctor will tell you what to watch for to identify infection and when to report it after any procedure or surgery you may have during your treatment. Patients that develop and infection after a stent (called **cholangitis**) may require antibiotics and sometimes replacement of the stent.

Endoscopic retrograde cholangiopancreatography (ERCP)

A procedure in which an endoscope (camera) is inserted into the stomach through the esophagus to visualize the performance of various procedures, including placing a stent or metal tube in bile ducts to relieve jaundice.

Stent

A piece of plastic or metal that is used to open a collapsed opening in the body.

Cholangitis

Infection involving symptoms such as fever, shaking chills, severe abdominal pain, and worsening jaundice. This infection is sometimes caused after bacteria are introduced into the bile duct system after an ERCP or percutaneous intervention to relieve jaundice.

15. How is extrahepatic bile duct cancer diagnosed?

During a physical examination, you may look jaundiced and your doctor may find that your liver is firm or enlarged. Imaging tests, such as an ultrasound, can show where the cancer is and the level of obstruction in the bile duct. A CT scan can provide the same information with a clearer assessment as to the extent of the cancer, and can determine whether or not the cancer is operable.

It is imperative that the CT scan includes the chest, abdomen, and pelvis, with particular focus on the area of the bile ducts next to the liver. You may need a procedure called an endoscopic retrograde cholangiopancreatography (ERCP). This is a procedure that is performed by passing a thin, lighted tube (an endoscope) through the mouth and down to the first part of the small intestine (the duodenum). A smaller tube is then passed through the endoscope and dye is injected so that clear pictures of all the branches of the biliary system can be taken. During the procedure, the physician may also take a biopsy of the duct to confirm the cancer diagnosis, and a stent may also be placed to relieve any blockage found. This should provide relief if you have had symptoms from blockage.

Many centers favor first doing a very specialized form of MRI called a **magnetic resonance cholangiopancreatography (MRCP)** prior to the ERCP to help visualize the details of the bile duct, the cancer, and the obstruction.

While your doctors will make every attempt to obtain an adequate biopsy, there is a chance the cancer cells won't show, and you may need a repeat biopsy and surgery to secure the diagnosis.

16. What are the symptoms of gallbladder cancer?

Gallbladder cancer can present without symptoms and is sometimes found at the time of gallbladder removal for another reason (e.g., suspected gallstones). However, some patients may experience abdominal pain on the upper right side of their abdomen where the gallbladder is located. Your doctor may feel a mass or a tumor at the site. In more advanced situations, you might have an enlarged liver or a distended abdomen because of the collection of fluid, a condition called ascites (see Question 88). You may even appear jaundiced (see Question 84). Your doctor might also order blood work

It is imperative that the CT scan includes the chest, abdomen, and pelvis, with particular focus on the area of the bile ducts next to the liver.

Magnetic resonance cholangiopancreatography (MRCP)

A specialized form of MRI performed before an ERCP that helps visualize the details of the bile duct, cancer, and obstruction.

Anemia

A condition marked by a lowering of the red blood cell count, resulting in fatigue.

Tumor marker

A protein that is secreted into the blood. Tumor markers may be elevated in biliary cancers. Tumor markers that are important in biliary cancers include CEA, CA 19-9, and AFP.

to further diagnose the gallbladder cancer. Increased liver enzymes, **anemia**, a low protein level, or elevated **tumor markers** (proteins that are secreted into the blood that may be elevated in biliary cancers) are all abnormalities that need further investigation.

17. How is gallbladder cancer diagnosed?

Gallbladder cancer is often diagnosed incidentally at the time of gallbladder removal for what are thought to be gallstones. Almost half of the cases of gallbladder cancer are found this way and, unfortunately, almost all of those cases show metastatic gallbladder cancer by that time.

Performing an ultrasound is an excellent way to help assess gallbladder tumors. Ultrasound is a very safe and simple test during which a doctor or radiology technician will apply a probe over your gallbladder area and generate pictures of the gallbladder, similar to visualizing a developing baby in the womb of a pregnant woman. Ultrasound has its limitations though, such as in conditions of inflammation that can be associated with the presence of gallstones, that can cause visualizing the cancer to become more difficult. Because of this, your doctor may order a CT scan to further assess the gallbladder as well as the extent of the cancer.

Performing an ultrasound is an excellent way to help assess gallbladder tumors.

18. What is a pathology report of a biopsy?

Pathology report

A medical report that describes important features of a disease. With cancer, it describes the type of cancer and degree of differentiation, both of which may affect the prognosis.

The **pathology report** describes important features of the cancer—specifically, the type of cancer (e.g., adenocarcinoma or squamous cell carcinoma). It also describes the degree of differentiation (how like or unlike the cancer cells are to normal biliary tissue). This will influence the treatment and prognosis. For patients who have undergone surgical removal of the cancer (e.g., gallbladder and/or liver resection), the pathology report also describes several other features of the cancer:

- The edges (margins) of the cancer are described, specifically whether there is normal tissue surrounding the cancer on all sides. If not, microscopic cancer cells may be left behind.

- The number of lymph nodes removed is listed along with the number of lymph nodes found to have cancer cells.

- The depth of tumor through the wall of the gallbladder or the bile duct.

- Whether or not blood vessel (**vascular**) or nerve (**perineural**) invasion is present.

- The size of the tumor.

- The extent of tumor involvement.

Vascular
Concerning the blood vessels.

Perineural
Concerning the nerves.

All of this information is important in determining the prognosis and what additional treatment will be recommended.

19. What is cancer staging, and why is it relevant?

Cancer staging refers to the extent of the cancer. Most cancers, including biliary cancers, are staged with the TNM (tumor, node, and metastasis) classification.

The T refers to different things depending on the tumor type. This is reflective of the pattern of spread of each

Cancer staging
A system of measurement that describes the extent of the cancer, measuring tumor type (T), involvement of lymph nodes (N), and whether the cancer has metastasized (M).

cancer. In the case of an intrahepatic cholangiocarcinoma, T refers to the tumor size and involvement of blood vessels and/or other organs or structures. In terms of an extrahepatic bile duct cancer, the T refers to the extent of the cancer and involvement of other organs or structures. When referring to gallbladder cancer, the wall of the gallbladder is made of several layers, including muscle, so the T in regards to gallbladder cancer refers to the depth of the cancer and how many layers are involved.

N refers to whether lymph nodes are (N1) or are not (N0) involved. M refers to the presence (M1) or absence (M0) of metastasis, or the spread of the cancer beyond the local area.

The importance of staging relates to the outcome of the cancer. As with other cancers, the earlier the stage of biliary cancer, the better the outcome.

The T, N, and M grades are grouped together into a stage that ranges from Stage I to IV. Generally, Stages I and II refer to cancers that are surgically removable. Stage III implies a locally advanced disease that has not spread or metastasized but is not operable. Stage IV refers to metastatic cancer, or cancer that has spread to other parts of the body (e.g., the liver, inner lining of the abdominal cavity, or the lungs). The importance of staging relates to the outcome of the cancer. As with other cancers, the earlier the stage of biliary cancer, the better the outcome.

20. How is staging performed?

Staging is best performed using a CT scan, an MRI, or a combination of the two. Imaging should include the chest, as biliary cancers may spread or metastasize to the lung.

In the case of extrahepatic bile duct cancer (see Question 15), an MRCP can provide detailed information on the bile duct anatomy and involvement without the need for an invasive ERCP when jaundice is not present. However, direct **cholangiography** (a technique performed by puncturing the skin and passing a small tube across the liver into the bile ducts under X-ray guidance) or ERCP is typically performed for patients with jaundice and/or inoperable cancer to relieve symptoms of bile duct blockage (jaundice, itching, malaise).

Cholangiography

A technique involving puncturing the skin and passing a small tube through the liver and into the bile ducts under X-ray guidance.

In certain cases, a physician may feel that surgery is the best way to complete staging. This surgery may include removal of all or part of the tumor. Sometimes performing a laparoscopic or "keyhole"-type surgery to evaluate the inner lining of the abdominal cavity for spread of the cancer does this. Laparoscopic surgery is often performed as an outpatient procedure or may require a hospital stay. If it does require a hospital stay, it is typically shorter than that required by an open operation.

PART FOUR

Coping with the Diagnosis

How long do people with biliary cancer live?

What is palliative care?

Should a patient get a second opinion?

More . . .

21. How long do people with biliary cancer live?

This is a difficult question and no simple answer is available. The life expectancy of someone diagnosed with biliary cancer is directly related to the stage of the cancer, the patient's level of well being at diagnosis, and what type of treatment is offered. For example, people who have operable and localized cholangiocarcinoma fare significantly better than patients with metastatic disease. Your doctor can estimate your survival based on how large groups of patients with cancer similar to yours have done in the past. However, even experienced physicians often cannot accurately determine how one particular patient may fare.

Building a close relationship with your physicians is important in helping to deal with fears that may occur when diagnosed with cancer. Your doctors should be in a position to recommend the best approach of therapy based on the stage of the disease.

Gary Rosen's comment:

As with most folks today, once I had a diagnosis, I went on the Internet to "learn" about my condition. Biliary cancer is not insignificant, and everything that I read was depressing. When I met with Dr. Abou-Alfa, I listened to his assessment and discussed treatment, but I never asked what my life expectation would be. My attitude was then, and is now, that this is an "extreme inconvenience," but I still have things to do in my life. Four and a half years later, I get my treatments every other week and carry on with my life.

22. What is supportive care?

The diagnosis of biliary cancer may have a significant impact on a patient's level of well being. The cancer, along with the treatments, may make the body weak and tired. In addition to the cancer itself, other concerns, including nutrition and pain control, might be present. This is not to understate the psychological, social, and financial impacts that a diagnosis of cancer may have on patients and their family and friends. Someone who is working and is found to have biliary cancer might have his or her lifestyle severely affected.

Although this may seem very discouraging, most doctors believe that a multifaceted support team approach can help alleviate many of the impacts of a cancer diagnosis. In addition to the **multidisciplinary care approach** (see Question 33), you also may need the help of pain specialists, nutritionists, psychiatrists, and social workers. A typical comprehensive cancer center has a team of several types of doctors and healthcare workers to fulfill this need. In addition, patient support groups and integrative or complementary medicine approaches may be helpful. **Integrative medicine** is a growing discipline that addresses the emotional, social, and spiritual needs of patients and their families as a whole. This helps to increase self-awareness and enhances a feeling of well being and may actualyl alleviate some anxieties and symptoms.

Multidisciplinary care

An approach in medicine that involves a team of healthcare workers, including surgeons, medical oncologists, interventional radiologists, radiation oncologists, and other specialists specific to what's being treated.

Integrative medicine

A growing discipline in the medical field that addresses the medical needs, along with the emotional, social, and spiritual needs, of patients and their families.

23. Should a patient get a second opinion?

Patients who are diagnosed with cancer often obtain a second opinion. Most doctors encourage it, as the second opinion may provide the patient with additional information. You may actually receive conflicting opinions about treatment options and prognosis. This is because doctors may differ in their views regarding certain approaches of treatment that may not be clearly defined in the medical field. This is where implementation of the multidisciplinary care approach from the time of diagnosis is advantageous (see Question 33). This is a critical component of the medical care you should receive and may minimize your uncertainties regarding your cancer diagnosis and treatment. It is important to hear the opinions of a variety of of specialists. On the other hand, patients should try to avoid getting too many opinions or opinons of persons not educated in the appropriate fields. This can make things more confusing or even delay critical therapy.

It is important at least to hear an opinion from different types of specialists.

At the initial diagnosis, seeking a second opinion may be very valuable, because curative options, such as surgery, might not be available locally and a patient might need to seek medical care at a larger cancer center. In patients with very advanced cancer, the need for a second opinion may be less important. Some patients and their families might travel great distances to seek opinions and look for advanced or unproven treatments. In this instance, most doctors recommend using common sense and good judgment to determine the need for second opinions.

Ultimately, your physician is in the best position to assess the usefulness of a second opinion, so it is important that you have an open and frank discussion about this topic together. Do not be surprised if your physician is the one who suggests a second opinion. In either instance, this is not a reflection of the inability of your physician to handle the current medical situation but rather a genuine effort to make you feel comfortable with the treatment plan that is recommended.

Gary Rosen's comment:

My first opinion was given by my local doctor, and my second was by Memorial. Biliary cancer is complex and rare, and most doctors, even local oncologists, only see a few cases in their careers. You really want to come to an institution like MSKCC where the doctors deal with multiple cases on a daily basis and are aware of the current research, clinical trials, and the most successful treatments.

24. Many people are volunteering different opinions. How should I handle that?

Undoubtedly, many people around you will express their concern and offer to help. Despite their good intentions, loved ones may offer advice that confuses, as it might contradict other advice that you have received or even your doctor's opinion. Most of the information that you will receive from your loved ones and acquaintances is based on personal experience or information gained from another person. Because not all cancers are the same, the information you receive may not be applicable to your particular case. Nonetheless, feel free to discuss any information or advice with your doctor so that it can be assessed objectively to see if any of it applies to your case.

It is also important to note that discussing your illness with others may infringe on your privacy, so you need to decide whom to discuss your diagnosis with and how much information to give them. Such discussions may be time consuming and even draining, both physically and mentally. They may have good intentions, but you are not obligated to take their feelings into consideration more than your own.

25. How should I manage my emotions now that I have been diagnosed with biliary cancer?

People differ in the way that they react to any adverse event in life. Some patients may have a better handle on a diagnosis of biliary cancer. Others may have a much more difficult journey, dealing with the new emotions, feelings, and stresses that come with a diagnosis of cholangiocarcinoma. Patients are not expected to understand their illness or to identify priorities that are important to them immediately.

Accepting the diagnosis of cancer might take a while, as some patients may have to first deal with their fear, denial, and anger. Patients fear cancer in general because of the uncertainty that comes with it. Patients are encouraged to discuss this fear with their doctors, because the more they learn about their disease, the more they will feel in control of the situation. Although patients might react with denial and anger, it is important to remember that these emotions are very normal. Patients might direct their anger against other people. It can be a very difficult situation, especially when those close close to the patient, such as family members, are dealing with their own anger and emotions. Patients and their loved ones are encouraged to express their fears, angers, and sadness, and to realize that, as they face the future, the need each other.

Guilt may also be present. Guilt is a very common and understandable emotion in these situations. The possibility of leaving your loved ones, being left behind, and/ or coping with the past and future, are all facets of guilt and fear.

Guilt is a very common and understandable emotion in these situations.

Another common emotion of a cancer patient is depression, which is a normal and sometimes expected reaction to the acceptance of a new diagnosis of biliary cancer. Patients should be aware of its signs and symptoms because many of the signs of depression can be confused with the signs of the cancer itself, such as a loss of appetite and a decreased level of energy. Fatigue is a common symptom of depression, and may be misinterpreted as a symptom of the cancer or its therapy. Nonetheless, even the subtle feeling of being depressed should be shared with the physician so that supportive action can be taken.

Patients are encouraged to have an open discussion with their caregivers, and to seek help for any concerning feelings. In many instances, professional help from a psychiatrist, social worker, or even medications might be needed, and this should be accepted as an integral part of the healing process. Some patients may wish to seek out spiritual support from priests or ministers from various faiths. Patient representatives may be able to help put these feelings in context and support patients and their families through a difficult time period.

Patients are encouraged to have an open discussion with their caregivers, and to seek help for any concerning feelings.

Gary's comment:

This is a serious condition, and you're in for an uphill battle. However, you should look at this battle as one you are eager to fight. I have my moments when I think about my situation, but then I shift my thoughts to my job (yes, I'm still working 5 days a week) or whatever the task at hand is and don't allow myself to get caught up in self-pity. Keeping normal life routines can be challenging, but that is my goal. It helps keep me from focusing on my condition and gives me a positive outlook.

Though it may seem a bit odd, guilt also enters into this situation. I feel guilty knowing that my family is dealing with my condition and that they are suffering emotionally more than me. That is more incentive for keeping a positive outlook in order to help them cope.

26. What insurance and financial concerns does a patient need to address after a diagnosis of biliary cancer?

Organized and well-documented information might save a great deal of trouble later on.

This is an important aspect of today's medical care. Health care is expensive, and patients with biliary cancer might need to stop working, at least temporarily, which can affect their insurance coverage. After being diagnosed with biliary cancer, you need to start collecting information about the health coverage options you have. Does your health insurance company provide only in-network coverage, limiting your choices to just the different providers and/or hospitals that the insurance company has an agreement with? Or do you have out-of-network coverage, allowing you to seek medical care wherever you wish? You should make sure that all of your insurance premiums are paid and that all information is up-to-date. Additionally, be sure to document all contacts with your insurance company. Organized and well-documented information might save a great deal of trouble later on. Most clinics and hospitals have a patient financial services department. It is important to establish contact with such a department to understand your rights and obligations.

Based on the severity of the illness or the extent of the treatment prescribed, you might be required to take a sick leave or even be placed on disability. This can be done through your employer or a disability policy through your insurance agency, which may already be in place.

The government also has several programs that may help you. These are divided into two distinct categories. The first category is made up of programs that are not based on income or financial means. This includes **Medicare**, which is for persons above 65 years of age. Details about the program may be found on the official website, www.medicare.gov. Two additional programs in this category are **social security** (*www.ssa.gov*), which is also for patients above 65 years of age, and **social security disability** (*www.ssa.gov*), which is for disabled workers and their family and is based on their disabled status and their prior contribution to the program. U.S. veterans also might seek veterans' benefit through the Department of Veterans Affairs (*www.va.gov*).

The second category consists of a single program, **Medicaid**. Medicaid is available if a patient does not have the means to obtain health care, he or she may seek government support through Medicaid. Details about the program can be found at *www.medicaid.gov*.

Medicare

Government-provided health insurance available to people over the age of 65.

Social security

Government-provided financial assistance available to people over the age of 65 or who earn little or no income.

Social security disability

Government-provided financial assistance available to people who earn little or no income due to a disability.

Medicaid

Government-provided health insurance available to people who are unable to receive health insurance another way.

Biological therapy

A type of therapy that operates like a key against a specific cancer target or a lock. While some therapies, or keys, are specific to certain cancers, or locks, others may have an effect on many different targets, like a master key.

Targeted therapy

Medication that specifically targets the cells needed for cancer growth.

Similarly, you need to verify if you have a medication coverage plan. New cancer therapies and other supportive medications (e.g., anti-nausea medicines) are available in pill form. These pills are not supported by your medical insurance and are either paid by a medication coverage plan or out of pocket. Some of these, such as **biological** and **targeted therapies,** are extremely expensive. Understanding your coverage plan and benefits early may give you a chance to identify and rectify any limiting issues, so your cancer therapy isn't delayed. Make sure to ask, as you may not necessarily be aware of all resources that are available to you.

PART FIVE

Treatment

What treatment options are available
for intrahepatic cholangiocarcinoma?

What determines whether a bile duct cancer
can be removed?

What is multidisciplinary care?

More...

Liver resection

Surgery that removes part of the liver.

Hepatectomy

Removal of the liver.

Radiofrequency ablation (RFA)

A procedure that involves the insertion of a metal probe into tissue to heat it up in order to kill the tissue.

Hepatic artery embolization

A procedure that involves the injection of substances into the blood vessels of a tumor.

Chemotherapy

The use of medication to kill or stop the growth of cancerous cells.

Chemoembolization

A treatment plan that uses both chemotherapy and hepatic artery embolization.

Radioactive bead ablation

A procedure in which small beads that contain radioactive material, known as microspheres, are injected into the blood vessels that directly feed the tumor in order to kill it.

27. Which treatment options are available for intrahepatic cholangiocarcinoma?

Several treatment options are available for patients with cholangiocarcinoma. In general, the most effective therapy is to remove the cancer. This can be done in one of two ways. One method is to remove the part of the liver that contains the tumor. This is called a **liver resection** or partial **hepatectomy**. The other option is to remove your entire liver and replace it with a new liver. This is called a liver transplantation.

If the tumor cannot be removed but is limited to the liver, your doctors may recommend a **radiofrequency ablation (RFA)**. This is performed by inserting a metal probe into the tumor and then heating it up, killing the cancer cells. Your doctor may also recommend a **hepatic artery embolization**, a procedure in which the blood vessels that feed your tumor are cut off by injecting blocking material into them. **Chemotherapy** may be used in conjunction with hepatic artery embolization, a treatment called **chemoembolization**.

Your doctors may also recommended you have a **radioactive bead ablation**. This is a procedure in which very small beads containing radioactive material, known as microspheres, are injected into the blood vessels feeding your tumor, killing the tumor. These procedures are usually performed by interventional radiologists, although they are sometimes carried out by surgeons.

You may not be a candidate for any of the previously listed procedures if your tumor has not responded to them previously, your tumor has spread to too many sites within the liver, or your cancer has metastasized outside of the liver. If this is the case, **systemic therapy** is generally considered the most appropriate treatment. Systemic therapy usually consists of chemotherapy that is given intravenously. Once in the blood stream, the chemotherapy agents can travel almost anywhere in the body, attacking the cancer cells wherever they are lodged. Your chemotherapy may consist of approved drugs, newer agents that are under investigation. This is called a **clinical trial** or study. The combination of the drugs **gemcitabine** and **cisplatin** is considered a standard option for inoperable biliary cancers. You may also be asked to join a clinical trial that is studying biological therapy, chemotherapy, or a combination of the two approaches.

Gary's comment:

I was not a candidate for any of the surgical options, so I began with gemcitabine and cisplatin. Like most folks, I had heard about the horrible side effects from chemotherapy, and my expectations were not good. In reality is that the medications they gave me to counter the side effects were extremely effective. While I was getting my treatments, I would usually eat lunch and watch a movie. After 2 years, my treatment changed to intrahepatic infusion pump (see Question 69), and now the procedure only takes about 45 minutes — too quick for lunch and a movie. My new treatment makes my nose run, and I will feel a bit "off" for a couple of days after, but it hasn't been anything but a nuisance. Keep moving and carry on!

28. What treatment options are available for extrahepatic bile duct cancers?

The treatment of operable biliary cancers requires expert surgeons who typically act as part of a team in major cancer centers. Surgical treatment will likely require

TREATMENT

Systemic therapy

A type of treatment that can attack the cancer throughout the entire body, no matter where it is or it might go.

Clinical trial

A research study that seeks to test new treatment options for a disease.

Gemcitabine

A chemotherapy drug that causes cell death by changing the DNA of the cancer cells.

Cisplatin

A chemotherapy drug that causes cell death by changing the DNA of the cancer cells.

100 QUESTIONS & ANSWERS ABOUT BILIARY CANCER

Recurrence
The return of a cancer after it has been treated and gone into remission.

removal of part of the liver to help reduce the chance of **recurrence**.

In the case of a tumor that has spread to beyond the local area, systemic therapy given intravenously would be the recommended treatment. Chemotherapy drugs can travel almost anywhere in the body and attack the cancer cells wherever they may be. As with intrahepatic biliary cancer, chemotherapy may involve the administration of approved drugs or new agents that are under investigation (this is called a clinical trial or study). The combination of gemcitabine and cisplatin is considered a standard option in this setting. You may also be asked join a clinical trial that is studying biological therapy, chemotherapy, or a combination of the two.

29. Which treatment options are available for gallbladder cancer?

If it is possible, the best treatment option for gallbladder cancer is surgery. After an inadvertent removal of a cancerous gallbladder during a routine gallbladder surgery for possible gallstones, a further surgery may be undertaken to remove the surrounding tissue and any lymph nodes near to where the gallbladder was.

Chemotherapy drugs can travel almost anywhere in the body and attack the cancer wherever it may be.

In the case of a tumor that has spread to beyond the local area, systemic therapy given intravenously would then be the appropriate treatment, similar to cholangiocarcinoma and extrahepatic biliary cancers. Chemotherapy drugs can travel almost anywhere in the body and attack the cancer wherever it may be. Chemotherapy may involve administration of approved drugs or new agents that are under investigation (this is called a clinical trial or study). As with intra- and extrahepatic biliary cancer combination of gemcitabine and cisplatin is considered a standard option in this setting. You may also be asked a clinical trial that is studying biological therapy, chemotherapy, or a combination of the two. Each of these treatments is discussed in detail elsewhere.

30. What determines whether a cholangiocarcinoma can be removed?

Several factors determine whether a cholangiocarcinoma can be removed. These include your general health condition, the condition of the cancer-free portion of your liver, and the distribution of the cancer and its relationship to vital structures in the liver including major blood vessels and bile ducts.

You must be in adequate general health in order to tolerate general anesthesia and a major operation such as liver resection. For instance, if a patient has a weak heart, an attempt at a liver resection may not be advisable as it may be too dangerous. Additionally, the noncancerous part of your liver must be healthy enough to tolerate a liver resection. The liver is a unique organ because it can regrow after part of it is removed. The liver is divided into right and left lobes and further divided into eight individual segments. Up to six of these segments (roughly 80%) of a healthy liver can typically be removed. Remarkably, the liver regrows within several weeks after removal, and normal liver function is restored within 4 weeks of a liver resection.

You must be in adequate general health in order to tolerate general anesthesia and a major operation such as liver resection.

However, some patients with cholangiocarcinoma have cirrhosis of the liver (underlying liver malfunction) and may be able have only a small percentage of the liver safely removed. Because patients with advanced

Varices

Enlarged blood vessels at risk of major bleeding.

Portal vein embolization

A procedure in which a substance is injected into the portal vein on the tumor to decrease blood flow to it, stimulating the other side of the liver to grow.

Portal vein

The vein that supplies blood to the liver.

cirrhosis often have **varices** (enlarged blood vessels at risk of major bleeding) or have blood that has trouble clotting, most patients with advanced cirrhosis cannot undergo any liver resection due to a high risk of bleeding to death during or shortly after the operation. These patients can also die from liver failure in the first few weeks after liver resection. While their liver may function well enough for everyday living, it may not be able to handle the stress of a liver resection.

In some patients, the portion of the liver that can remain following the operation is judged to be insufficient in size. Depending on the degree of cirrhosis and the amount expected to be removed, your surgeon may elect to grow a portion of your liver prior to the operation. This can be done using a procedure called **portal vein embolization**. During this procedure, an interventional radiologist injects a blocking material into the **portal vein** on the side of your tumor to decrease blood flow to that portion of your liver. This stimulates the side of your liver that is not affected to grow, reducing the percentage of your liver that is being removed. Having a large portion of your liver left behind following the operation will make it easier for you to recover.

Additional factors considered when planning the surgery are the extent of the cancer within the liver and how many of the vital structures of the liver are affected by it. Most patients who are treated with liver resection have a single tumor. Typically, doctors do not suggest resection as an option for patients with multiple tumors in their liver, as the cancer may recur quickly.

31. What determines whether my bile duct cancer can be removed by surgery?

Since the resection of bile duct cancer is a major operation that requires general anesthesia, you need to be adequate general health in order for it to be considered. If you are eligible, the objectives of surgical management of bile duct cancer include both complete removal of tumor and establishing adequate biliary drainage. Unfortunately, most bile duct tumors are found to be already extensive and inoperable. Because open surgery is an extensive operation that carries risks, your surgeon is most likely to start with a laparoscopy procedure first to determine if the cancer can be removed or not (see Question 35).

During a surgery to remove cancer from the biliary system, you may be found to require surgical removal of a part of the liver if there is concern about it being affected cancerous or to help prevent the cancer from recurring. Thus, the noncancerous part of your liver must be deemed healthy enough for you to undergo a liver resection. You will likely be jaundiced with this type of cancer (see Question 84), and may need a biliary drainage (see Question 85) before you go to surgery.

If your bile duct cancer began nearby the small intestine and the pancreas, the extent of the cancer, both locally and in the blood vessels, may determine if the cancer can be surgically removed or not. If the cancer is operable, a surgery called a **Whipple procedure** may be performed. The Whipple procedure involves the removal of the lower part of the bile duct, the gallbladder, the head of the pancreas, and part of the small bowel (duodenum). It also reconnects the pancreas to the stomach and the bowel to the pancreas and stomach.

Unfortunately, many bile duct tumors are found to be already extensive and inoperable.

Whipple procedure

A procedure that involves the removal of the lower part of the bile duct, the gallbladder, the head of the pancreas, and the duodenum, and reconnects the pancreas to the stomach and the bowel to the pancreas and stomach.

TREATMENT

32. What factors determine whether a gallbladder cancer can be removed or not?

As mentioned in Question 29, discovering cancer during a routine laparoscopic gallbladder surgery is a common way for gallbladder cancer to be diagnosed. If the surgeon recognizes this at the time of surgery, an appropriate approach may be to abort the surgery and refer you to a specialized surgeon to have a more extensive surgery that ensures the removal of all cancerous and surrounding tissue. However, it is more common for the cancer to not be discovered until the pathology report has been finalized.

Typically, if a patient with gallbladder cancer has jaundice, this indicates that the cancer is advanced and generally an operation to remove the cancer is not possible.

In either case, the factors that determine complete resectability include the extent of the cancer locally and or whether there has been more distant spread of the cancer. This can often be clarified by updated imaging (CT scan, MRI, or PET scan) and by laparoscopy ("keyhole" or small incision surgery to evaluate the inner lining of the abdominal cavity). Additionally, your medical condition at that time will also be a critical factor in determining your fitness for surgery. Typically, if a patient with gallbladder cancer has jaundice, this indicates that the cancer is advanced and generally an operation to remove the cancer is not possible. In this latter setting, arrangements will typically be made to relieve the jaundice with either a stent or a drain before starting chemotherapy.

33. What is multidisciplinary care?

Biliary cancers are very complex diseases that require the input of multiple specialists to ensure the best treatment plan. This multidisciplinary team typically consists of **heptobiliary surgeons, medical oncologists, interventional radiologists, radiation oncologists, hepatologists**, and, occasionally, **gastroenterologists**. Depending on what other services are offered at your medical facility, this team may include other types of specialists, as well. For example, a surgeon and an interventional radiologist may need to confer on how to ensure regrowth of your liver after surgery (see Question 30).

Surgeons and, more specifically, hepatobiliary surgeons, who specialize in biliary-, liver-, and pancreatic-cancer surgeries, will decide whether your tumor can be removed. A medical oncologist is a cancer doctor who specializes in the use of systemic or medical treatments for your cancer, which includes chemotherapy and biological therapies. A gastroenterologist may be involved in the diagnosis of your cancer and in addressing any blockage of the bile ducts, similar to an interventional radiologist, and can also assist with making a diagnosis or relieving blockages.

As you can imagine, many medical situations are not straightforward, and there is value to having a multidisciplinary assessment. Having your case discussed in an open format where specialists give their opinions about the best approach to treating your cancer will undoubtedly help you receive the most appropriate treatment. It is important to understand that physicians are used to this format of meetings, and are usually open to critique and differing opinions. This approach emanates from their basic understanding of the complexity of the human body, diseases, and medicine, and that there can be more than one answer to a problem. Do not hesitate to ask or support your doctor to have your case presented at a multidisciplinary forum.

Heptobiliary surgeons

Surgeons who specialize in operating on biliary and liver cancers.

Medical oncologist

A doctor whose focus is in diagnosing cancer, managing it, and treating it using methods including chemotherapy, targeted therapy, and biological therapy.

Interventional radiologist

A physician who utilizes minimally invasive, image-guided procedures to diagnose and treat cancers.

Radiation oncologist

A physician who uses ionizing radiation to treat cancer.

Hepatologists

Physicians who focus on the liver and its ailments.

Gastroenterologists

Physicians whose practice focuses on the gastrointestinal tract.

TREATMENT

Gary's comment:

The doctors at MSKCC have multidisciplinary teams, and I know that Dr. Abou-Alfa, my medical oncologist, occasionally discusses my case with members of the team to get their opinions on an option that he may be considering. This gives me confidence that I'm getting the best treatment because each of the different disciplines have different options and experiences and pooling their knowledge is a good thing for me.

34. What preparations are made before a surgery?

After the patient and doctor decide that a surgery should be undertaken, certain precautionary steps will be taken. Older patients or those with certain preexisting medical problems may need to see a general physician, a cardiologist (heart specialist), or a pulmonologist (lung specialist) to determine whether they are fit enough to undergo an operation. During this evaluation, they may be asked to undergo certain special tests, such as a stress test or an **echocardiogram** to assess heart function.

Next, the patient will undergo what is called **preadmission testing**. This testing may include blood tests, an **electrocardiogram** (a method of tracing the heart), and a chest X-ray, and is standard practice before undergoing general anesthesia. Often, the patient will meet their anesthesiologist. In most cases, patients will be admitted to the hospital on the day of the operation. If special medical circumstances exist, a patient may be admitted to the hospital for several days before the operation. Depending on the location of the tumor, the surgeon may have the patient take medication to clean out the intestines before surgery.

Echocardiogram

An ultrasound of the heart.

Preadmission testing

Standard testing before undergoing anesthesia that involves blood tests, an electrocardiogram, and a chest X-ray.

Electrocardiogram

An imaging test that produces tracings of the heart.

On the morning of surgery, you are not allowed to eat or drink, and your physician will have told you whether to take your normal medications with a sip of water. You will be asked to arrive at the hospital several hours before the scheduled time of the operation, even as early as 6 am so that everything is ready in time for the surgery. Most surgeons begin operating early in the morning. You will be asked to get undressed and to put on a hospital gown. Patients are generally kept in a comfortable waiting area called the holding area until the operating room is ready. In some hospitals, families may be able to stay with the patient during this time. Different doctors, nurses, assistants, and other hospital staff will each ask you for your name, your medical history, the intended surgical procedure, and your allergies. Such repetition may become annoying, but it is done to ensure your safety and is required to ensure that the correct patient is undergoing the correct operation.

When the operating room is ready, the patient is usually taken to it. There, the patient will meet several nurses, surgical assistants, an anesthesiologist, and the surgeon. The operating room is often chilly, but you will be covered with several blankets during the operation. An intravenous (IV) drip will be inserted into your arm now if one was not inserted while you were in the holding area. Fluids will be delivered through this IV to keep you hydrated during surgery. Anesthetic and other medications will also be administered through the IV as needed. You will lie flat on your back upon a table and a mask will be placed on your face through which you will be asked to breathe. Anesthetic will then be pumped through this mask until you drift into a deep sleep or unconsciousness.

35. What happens during a surgery?

After you are asleep, any hair on your stomach will be shaved before being washed with soap. Generally, a small tube, called a Foley catheter, will be placed into the bladder so that the amount of urine can be closely monitored. A larger IV line may be placed into your neck to give additional fluids and/or medications that might be needed for support through the operation. Your surgeon will discuss this with you before the operation.

In some circumstances, the surgeon may decide to perform a laparoscopy first. In a laparoscopy, a few small incisions (less than an inch) are made in order to insert a scope and other medical instruments into the abdomen. Specifically, the surgeon is looking to see whether the cancer is more advanced or has spread outside of the liver, which sometimes cannot be seen on the radiologic tests that were done before surgery. If you have the liver condition cirrhosis (see Question 6), the surgeon will also determine how bad it is and decide if the surgery should continue.

Once an incision has been made, your surgeon will determine whether your tumor can actually be removed. While your tumor may have appeared to be removable in the CT scan or MRI leading up to the surgery, the surgeon may now find that your tumor cannot be removed. This can be for several reasons, including spread of the tumor outside the liver in the case of cholangiocarcinoma, inability to remove the tumor safely from vital structures (e.g., due to risk of major bleeding or bile duct injury), or spread of the tumor to adjacent structures or organs.

36. How extensive is the surgery?

If the tumor is removable, the surgeon will continue with the procedure. The extent of surgery will depend on the type and size of the tumor you have. As part of the operation for cholangiocarcinoma, the surgeon may have to remove your gallbladder to expose other structures of the liver. In surgery for bile duct cancer close to the liver, your surgeon will most likely remove a part of your liver to ensure a full removal of the cancer. On the other hand, if your bile duct cancer is closer to the duodenum and involves the very end of the bile duct that travels through the pancreas before reaching the duodenum, your surgeon will perform what is called a Whipple procedure. In a Whipple procedure, your surgeon will remove the head of the pancreas, part of the duodenum, and part of the bile duct. The surgeon will also reconnect the bile duct to a different part of the small bowel, connect a loop of bowel to the stomach, and reconnect the pancreatic duct to the bowel. While operating on gallbladder cancer, your surgeon may remove part of your liver and any nearby lymph nodes due to the potential spread of the cancer to those areas.

If you are having your gallbladder removed by laparoscopy through a small incision and cancer is found incidentally (i.e., before the pathology information is available), the surgeon may stop the surgery and refer you to an expert for an appropriate surgery. This usually involves the removal of a part of liver and any nearby lymph nodes.

In surgery for bile duct cancer close to the liver, your surgeon will most likely remove a part of your liver to ensure a full removal of the cancer.

Similarly, if your gallbladder was already removed and your cancer was discovered on pathology, you may well need another surgery to perform an optimal cancer operation. This will involve the removal of a part of your liver and any nearby lymph nodes and is the best chance of reducing the risk of recurrence.

37. What happens in the hospital after surgery?

The main risk within the first 12 hours of surgery is bleeding at the site of surgery.

After the operation, you will be taken to a recovery room for close observation. The main risk within the first 12 hours of surgery is bleeding at the site of surgery. Rarely, a patient may need to undergo an emergency operation to control bleeding. Depending on the hospital, you will stay in a highly monitored setting for anywhere from half a day to several days before being transferred to a regular patient floor. Overall, you can expect to be in the hospital for between 5 and 10 days. If everything goes well, you should be able to sit in a chair and, in many cases, walk the day after your surgery. It often takes a few days before you are ready to eat again. A special intravenous pump is often used to provide pain medication. The nurse will explain how to use this type of pump.

38. What are the risks of surgery for biliary cancer?

Besides bleeding, another potential major complication from biliary cancer surgery is bile leakage. As your surgeon is operating on small bile ducts, there is a potential for leakage of bile that may be self contained and easily controlled. In some cases, however, the leakage can be extensive and build up in the abdomen and may require drainage by interventional radiologists. Bile can also become infected and require a course of antibiotics to eradicate the infection. Many patients will temporarily gain weight from the extra fluids that are pumped into the body around the time of the operation. You may notice that your ankles or your stomach are swollen from these extra fluids and that you have gained weight despite having fasted for several days.

Many patients will temporarily gain weight from the extra fluids that are pumped into the body around the time of the operation.

In some patients, the incision may not heal completely and actually open slightly. This may require special dressing changes while you are in the hospital and, in some cases, after you are discharged from the hospital as well. Fluid may begin to collect where the cancer was removed, and it may require drainage about a week later. This is usually done by an interventional radiologist or a gastroenterologist, and involves inserting a needle or a small drain to draw out the fluid. Other complications from major abdominal surgeries may include pneumonia, infection in your urine caused by the temporary tube that was placed into the bladder, or blood clots in the legs (deep vein thrombosis; DVT) or lungs (pulmonary emboli; PE). To protect against blood clots, you will be administered a blood thinner preventively via an injection into the skin of the abdomen or arm.

In the case of cholangiocarcinoma, some patients may have cirrhosis (liver malfunction), which puts them at an additional risk of complications from an operation. These patients may be more prone to gastrointestinal bleeding, which can arise from **gastritis**, an ulcer, or varices. Varices are veins in the esophagus or stomach that have dilated due to abnormally high pressure within a cirrhotic liver. Patients with cirrhosis also are at risk for ascites, which is the accumulation of fluid within the

Gastritis
Stomach irritation.

belly. Ascites is generally treated with diuretics ("water pills") that make you urinate more frequently.

After returning home, complete recovery will take 3 to 6 weeks. You will slowly regain your energy. You may not notice that improvement day by day, but over each week you will likely feel better. If you are not, then you should notify your doctor. With doctor approval, you can usually drive within a few weeks. By that point, you should be totally off pain medications. You should not do any heavy lifting for several months to avoid disrupting the incision. You should generally expect to regain your quality of life, although your doctor may discuss specific concerns related to your condition.

39. What is included in the pathology report from my surgery?

The pathology report from your surgery contains a lot of information. From it, the precise type and stage of the cancer can be determined. The written report, which can take about a week, will state the size and number of the tumors. In the case of gallbladder cancer, the pathologist will also determine how deep into the different layers of the gallbladder wall the cancer penetrated. If lymph nodes were removed, the report will state how many lymph nodes were removed and how many were affected by the cancer.

The pathologist will determine whether the surgeon achieved a negative margin of resection, or complete removal (i.e., the tumor was removed with a rim of normal tissue as a margin). If part of the liver was removed, the pathologist will also dissect the liver and look at the tumor under a microscope to determine whether it invaded any large or small blood vessels. If the cancer reached any blood vessels, you will have a higher rate recurrence. The last piece of information in the pathology report is the status of the noncancerous liver in case of liver resection. The pathologist will determine whether the liver shows any signs of damage or cirrhosis. If it does, the pathologist will give a grade for the degree of cirrhosis, scarring, or inflammation present in the liver.

40. Will I be cured after a surgery?

Generally surgical removal of biliary cancers is performed with the intent to cure. The best outcome is that all of the cancer is removed. While this is achieved in many patients, a majority will see recurrence. It is not understood why biliary cancers can recur after an apparently successful surgery, but it is assumed that it is related to the biology of the cancer and the fact that microscopic cells (which cannot be seen in scans) may have escaped prior to surgery. The best outcome possible in surgery is when the tumor is removed with clean margins and the lymph nodes are not involved.

For cholangiocarcinoma, your best chance of avoiding recurrence of the cancer is if the tumor was completely removed (negative margins), was of a small size, and did not spread to the lymph nodes or blood vessels. For bile duct cancers and gallbladder cancer, the chances of recurrence are less likely if the cancer does not extend through the gallbladder wall and into other organs and does not involve the lymph nodes. If the cancer returns, it is considered treatable, but is not a curable situation and typically complete eradication is not possible. Despite the lack of a guaranteed cure, you should undergo surgical removal of the cancer if advised to do so by your doctors.

It is not understood why biliary cancers can recur after an apparently successful surgery, but it is assumed that it is related to the biology of the cancer and the fact that microscopic cells (which cannot be seen in scans) may have escaped prior to surgery.

41. What are neoadjuvant and adjuvant therapies?

Adjuvant therapy

Treatment given after surgery to lessen the chance of the cancer's recurrence.

Neoadjuvant therapy

Treatment given before surgery to enhance the possibility of a successful surgery and to improve the outcome of the disease.

Radiation

A treatment that aims to kill cancer cells by using electromagnetic waves, which can be controlled and directed toward cancer cells.

Adjuvant therapy is treatment given after surgery to decrease the risk of recurrence. **Neoadjuvant therapy** is a similar type of treatment that is given before surgery to try and enhance the success of the operation and improve the outcome of the cancer.

Neoadjuvant therapy is an appealing strategy for several reasons:

- It offers definitive treatment of the cancer by opting patients who are extremely likely to develop metastatic disease early, sparing them a surgery that would be of no benefit to them.

- Chemotherapy and **radiation** may be somewhat more effective when given preoperatively, as they require well-oxygenated tissues for maximum effect and surgery tends to upset the blood supply.

- It is possible that combining preoperative chemotherapy and radiation may make a few "borderline resectable" patients operable.

- Patients can often receive a greater amount of preoperative therapy, as the delivery of postoperative therapy can be delayed due to slow postoperative recovery or other problems.

Currently, no definitive studies are available that compare preoperative with postoperative therapy to help decide which might be the better approach to manage biliary cancers.

Currently, no definitive studies are available that compare preoperative with postoperative therapy to help decide which might be the better approach to manage biliary cancers. For now, if the cancer is considered operable, surgery is the recommended first step.

42. Should I receive adjuvant chemotherapy and/or radiation therapy after surgery to prevent a recurrence of the tumor?

There is some evidence that adjuvant therapy using either chemotherapy alone or chemotherapy paired with radiation may help reduce the chances of biliary cancers recurring. However, this has not yet been proven in controlled or "randomized" studies, and there is no universal consensus as to whether to recommend treatment after surgery. If adjuvant therapy is offered as part of a clinical trial, you should consider it and may be encouraged by your doctor to take part in it.

It is imperative that you discuss with your doctor the pros and cons of receiving adjuvant therapy. If your tumor was unable to be completely removed during surgery, you most likely will be recommended additional treatment after you recover from the operation. Chemotherapy is typically recommended, but radiation will sometimes be suggested.

It is imperative that you discuss with your doctor the pros and cons of receiving adjuvant therapy.

43. If the tumor cannot be surgically removed now, can I have chemotherapy first and then undergo surgery?

Chemotherapy given before surgery with the intention of shrinking the tumor to allow for resection is called neoadjuvant therapy. There is no established standard of care for neoadjuvant treatment, meaning the value of this approach has not yet been proven in treating gallbladder cancers. Despite the lack of confirmed benefit, one scenario in which neoadjuvant therapy may be considered is if the bile duct cancer is localized. However, patients whose bile duct cancer is unresectable due to direct extension into the liver but has not metastasized to other organs may still be candidates for an experimental approach of neoadjuvant chemotherapy and radiation therapy followed by liver transplantation. This approach is recommended for a small number of patients with cholangiocarcinoma who fit the very stringent criteria required for the procedure to be effective. Such liver transplantations are done at a small number of specialized centers. It is best to discuss with your medical team whether this type of approach applies to you.

44. What happens if my biliary cancer returns?

Your doctor may discover that your tumor has returned based on a rise in tumor (cancer) markers (see Question 63), the results of radiologic tests, or the appearance of new symptoms. Several options are available if your cancer returns. If you have cholangiocarcinoma confined to the liver, you may be eligible for another liver surgery. Reoperation depends on similar factors listed in Question 30 and the extent of the first liver operation. The other treatment options for unresectable tumors include liver transplantation, tumor ablation, systemic therapy, liver-directed chemotherapy, clinical trials, and supportive care.

45. Can liver transplantation be performed for cholangiocarcinoma?

Liver transplantation can be considered in very special circumstances for patients with cholangiocarcinoma similar to patients with primary liver cancer. The aim is to have the entire liver—and the cancer contained within—removed as part of liver transplantation. This removes the tumor and any other areas of the liver that the cancer may have spread to. In a regular surgical operation, only the tumors visible to the naked eye of the surgeon are removed. This means that these cancerous, microscopic cells, if present, may be left behind and can result in tumor recurrence.

It is important to note that this approach is still in its early phases of development and is performed only at specific institutions or as a part of a clinical trial. If you and your doctor think this treatment option could work and wish to pursue it, you will need to be referred to one of these specialized institutions as early as possible.

46. Where do new livers for liver transplants come from?

A new liver may come from one of two sources. The first source is known as a **cadaveric transplant**. This is a liver that is obtained from a person whose brain has died but whose organs were donated during the brief period after the death of the brain in which they are still functional. Organs are only donated for transplantation with the consent of the family or of the deceased prior to death. An international organization called the United Network for Organ Sharing (UNOS) distributes the available organs to patients on a transplant waiting

Organs are only donated for transplantation with the consent of the family or of the deceased prior to death.

Cadaveric transplant

An organ for transplantation taken from a person who is brain-dead, but whose organs are still alive.

Living donor

A person who is still alive who chooses to donate an organ; this is typically a family member or friend of a patient.

list. Patients are given organs based on their degree of liver function and whether they have biological similarities, such as blood type and size, with the donor. The waiting time for a liver is variable, but could be as long as a few years, as there is a shortage of donor livers. As liver transplantation for biliary cancers is still considered experimental, you are not likely to have a high priority on the waiting list to receive a liver.

The other source is to remove a part of a liver from a **living donor**, often a family member or friend. This may be a more realistic and practical way to ensure obtaining a transplant for biliary caner, as it is faster than waiting on a transplant list. This can significantly extend the patient's life and prevent the patient from dying while on a waiting list for a cadaveric liver. Every effort is made to minimize potential complications to the donor, but liver resection is a major, potentially dangerous operation.

Again, the transplantation from either type of donor is still experimental for the treatment of biliary cancers. Your doctor should weigh in before you decide to join a waiting list or have someone volunteer to serve as a living donor.

47. What are the complications of liver transplantation?

Because of the technical complexity of performing a liver transplant and the immunologic aspects of receiving a new liver, several potential complications exist after liver transplantation:

- *Bleeding*: Like a liver resection, sometimes patients must undergo another operation to stop bleeding shortly after the original operation.

- *Liver blood vessels clotting or thrombosis*: Sometimes, the **hepatic artery**, one of the blood vessels that supply the liver with blood, can clot. Another operation may be needed to address this problem. In very bad cases, another liver transplant may have to be performed.

Hepatic artery

The artery that supplies blood to the liver.

- *Primary liver nonfunction or failure*: In some patients, the new liver fails to work properly for unknown reasons. Another liver may have to be transplanted immediately.

- *Biliary leak*: In some patients, bile can leak from the connection of the old bile duct to the new bile duct. This may require drainage of collected bile.

- *Rejection*: Your body may try to reject your new liver. Your doctor may adjust or change any immunosuppressants you are taking to avoid rejection. If your liver function becomes reduced and any symptoms of rejection, such as pain, fever, or flu-like symptoms, start to show, your doctor will have a liver biopsy performed to diagnose the extent of the rejection. It is very important to take your medications and to comply with frequent medical monitoring to avoid rejection, as it can lead to total liver failure.

- *Infection*: Infection can occur at anytime while you are taking immunosuppressants following the transplantation. Any sign of infection requires immediate medical attention, as even a minor one can be life threatening.

48. What is tumor ablation and can it be used for the treatment of cholangiocarcinoma?

Ablation is the destruction of a tumor without actually removing it. In some cases, the entire tumor can be destroyed, especially if the tumor is less than 3 cm in diameter. With larger tumors, it is more likely that a small part of the tumor will survive and begin to grow again.

Several techniques of ablation exist; hepatic artery embolization (with or without chemotherapy), alcohol injection, radiofrequency ablation, **cryotherapy**, and **irreversible electroporation (IRE)** are the most widely used. Some physicians will use them in combination. For instance, a hepatic artery embolization can be performed one day, followed by a radiofrequency ablation or an alcohol injection the next. Any of these various procedures can be repeated in the future if the tumor grows back. If you have multiple or large tumors, your doctors may elect to apply these procedures a few times within the first couple of months following your diagnosis.

Your multidisciplinary team will still need to discuss what the best approach for the treatment of your cancer is, however. For example, if there is spread of the cancer both inside and outside the liver, liver-directed therapies will typically be passed over in favor of chemotherapy or other medical treatments.

Gary Rosen's comment:

In my situation, chemotherapy has been the recommendation of the team. However, Dr. D'Angelica, my surgical oncologist, has assured me that there are options that may be considered in the event that the chemotherapy route becomes ineffective.

Ablation

The destruction of tissue internally, without removing it. Examples include alcohol injection, cryotherapy, irreversible electroporation, and hepatic artery embolization.

Cryotherapy

A procedure involving the insertion of a metal probe into tissue and freezing it, thereby destroying the tissue.

Irreversible electroporation (IRE)

A procedure that uses electricity to destroy tissue.

49. What is hepatic artery embolization and can it be used to treat cholangiocarcinoma?

Hepatic artery embolization is the injection of microscopic beads into the hepatic artery, clogging the blood vessels. Since a cholangiocarcinoma depends largely on blood supplied by the hepatic artery to survive, clogging it can destroy it. Clogging part of the hepatic artery is safe for your body, however, as your liver also receives blood from another vessel called the portal vein. Along with these particles, many doctors also inject a chemotherapy drug or use particles called drug-eluting beads, which have a chemotherapy agent attached to them. At the present, it is unclear whether adding a chemotherapy drug is more effective, and its usage will likely depend on your doctor's past experiences.

A specific type of radiologist called an interventional radiologist performs hepatic artery embolization. These radiologists are specialized in performing invasive procedures under X-ray guidance. The procedure is carried out in a hospital, and you will most likely be kept there for observation for a few days afterward. The procedure takes a couple of hours, requires only light sedation, and is carried out while you lie flat on a table. First, one of your legs (usually the right leg) is numbed with a tiny injection before a small tube is inserted into the femoral artery.

An X-ray machine is then positioned above you and is used to monitor the location of the small tube, which is passed through a large artery called the aorta and then into the hepatic artery, which feeds the liver. The tube is advanced further still into either the right or left branch of the hepatic artery. From there, the particles

At the present, it is unclear whether adding a chemotherapy drug is more effective, and its usage will likely depend on your doctor's past experiences.

can be released. In general, it is more desirable to selectively block the specific blood vessels that are supplying a tumor and to preserve the vessels going to the normal liver. At the end of the procedure, the tube is removed from the leg and you will lie flat for a further 4–6 hours to ensure that the wound heals and does not bleed.

The use of hepatic artery embolization for the treatment of cholangiocarcinoma is relatively uncommon. For the most part, hepatic artery embolization does not play a role in the treatment of gallbladder or extrahepatic bile duct cancers (see Question 52).

50. What are the side effects that may occur with hepatic artery embolization?

Embolization can cause a number of side effects, and most patients are admitted to the hospital for observation for 2–4 days following the procedure. In general, the magnitude of the side effects is proportional to the amount of tumor that is destroyed. If you have a large tumor that was completely embolized, you can expect to have a number of side effects due to the amount of dead tissue that results from the embolization. Dead tissue releases toxic substances into your blood stream, which can make you sick. Your liver may become irritated during the procedure, which can cause pain afterward. These symptoms can be controlled with medications. For the pain, you will typically receive IV pain medication, often via a **patient-controlled anesthesia (PCA) system**, which allows the patient to control how frequently the pain medication is delivered through the IV. You may not have an appetite for a few days following the procedure, and your doctor may recommend not eating until your other symptoms settle.

Patient-controlled anesthesia (PCA)

Pain medication that is delivered intravenously by the patient.

Following the embolization, you may experience fever coupled with an increase in the blood levels of liver enzymes. These side effects are collectively called **post-embolization syndrome** and typically last anywhere from a few days to several weeks. Rarely, embolization will cause a problem with heart or kidney function. Another unusual complication is the formation of an infection in the dead tumor tissue. This infection is known as an **abscess** and can be treated with antibiotics. In rare situations, you may need a drain placed into the infection.

The tube that was placed into the artery can also cause complications. Bleeding can occur at the puncture site in the groin and form a **pseudoaneurysm** or a large bruise called a **hematoma**. Additionally, the patient may require an operation to repair the blood vessel if it was damaged during the procedure.

51. What are radiofrequency ablation and cryotherapy, and can they be used for the treatment of cholangiocarcinoma?

Radiofrequency ablation and cryotherapy both destroy a tumor by exposing it to extreme temperatures via a metal probe. Radiofrequency ablation heats the tumor, whereas cryotherapy freezes it. They can only be used if there are a limited number of small to medium in size (less than 3–4 cm) tumors. Either procedure can be performed in a variety of ways. An interventional radiologist can place the probe percutaneously (meaning through the skin) in a procedure that requires sedation.

Either procedure can also be performed while the patient is under general anesthesia via a laparoscopy

Post-embolization syndrome

A condition that occurs following a hepatic artery embolization with symptoms such as fever and an increase in blood levels of liver enzymes. This syndrome usually resolves in a few days to several weeks.

Abscess

The development of an infection in dead tissue.

Pseudoaneurysm

A weakened sidewall of a blood vessel that can break or bleed easily.

Hematoma

A large bruise.

or an open laparotomy. Laparoscopy involves several small incisions in your abdomen, while an open laparotomy is performed through a cut in your abdomen. Your doctor will decide which of these methods is best for you based on the number, size, and location of your tumors. For instance, not all liver tumors can be reached percutaneously.

It is important to understand that not all tumors can be treated with radiofrequency ablation or cryotherapy. If a tumor is close to a main bile duct or a large blood vessel, the use of these techniques may be too risky. Some newer techniques for direct ablation, including microwave ablation and adding chemotherapy drugs to enhance radiofrequency ablation, are currently under study. Additionally, a new technique called IRE, which uses electricity to destroy the tumors, may be used for tumors located near bile ducts or major blood vessels. However, the value of IRE in the treatment of biliary and other cancers is under study and is not a routine approach at this time.

Some newer techniques for direct ablation, including microwave ablation and adding chemotherapy drugs to enhance radiofrequency ablation, are currently under study.

The use of radiofrequency ablation or cryotherapy for the treatment of cholangiocarcinoma is rare, as these tumors are uncommonly small or limited enough to allow successful interventions with these techniques. In general, if a cholangiocarcinoma is not considered surgically operable, it most likely requires systemic therapy. Similarly, it is unlikely that hepatic artery embolization plays a role in the case of bile duct cancer and gallbladder cancer, as any spread of these cancers to the liver implies the need for systemic therapy (see Question 52).

52. What is systemic therapy or chemotherapy?

Systemic therapy, or chemotherapy, is the use of **cytotoxic drugs** to kill or halt the growth of cancer cells ("cyto" derives from "cytology," or the study of cells). Chemotherapy agents are commonly given intravenously through a needle in the arm, though some drugs can be taken orally as pills and others can be administered directly into the liver (a process known as hepatic artery infusional chemotherapy). In IV chemotherapy, the drugs will be delivered throughout the body, or systemically, not just to selective sites. This carries the added advantage of treating the cancer at multiple sites if it has already spread to different sites inside or outside of liver.

"Chemotherapy" is a generic term that represents a vast assortment of different drugs, just as the term "antibiotics" encompasses a variety of agents that fight bacteria. Different chemotherapy drugs are used to combat specific cancers, and all have different potential side effects. It is important to note that chemotherapy is a constantly evolving science, and that the difficult experiences of patients in the past may not be a reality anymore, as new chemotherapies with fewer side effects and better supportive medications have been developed. How often chemotherapy is given depends on the drug or combination of drugs, as well as on the nature of the cancer and the patient's condition. Generally, intravenous chemotherapy is not given more than once per week.

TREATMENT

Cytotoxic drug

Medication that is used to kill or stop the growth of cells, especially cancerous cells.

It is important to note that chemotherapy is a constantly evolving science, and that the difficult experiences of patients in the past may not be a reality anymore, as new chemotherapies with fewer side effects and better supportive medications have been developed.

When determining the dosage of chemotherapy, doctors use something called the **body surface area (BSA)** to account for differences in patient size. BSA is calculated from the height and weight of a patient. You may notice that your chemotherapy dose is listed in mg/m². This is milligrams (amount of the drug) per square meter (this is your surface area). This method ensures that a tall or heavy patient would not be undertreated and also that a very short or thin patient would not be overtreated.

Body surface area

A measurement of size based on a person's height and weight.

53. Do I need to stay in the hospital to receive chemotherapy?

Most, if not all, chemotherapy is now given in the outpatient setting, and hospital admittance in order to receive chemotherapy is rare. Depending on where you are in your treatment and how well you are doing, you may need to see your medical oncology doctor on the day of your treatment. However, you will always have your blood work checked first. This is important, as many chemotherapy drugs affect your white and red blood cells and your platelets (see Question 54). If your blood work shows these cell levels to be in a safe range, you will receive your treatment that day.

Most, if not all, chemotherapy is now given in the outpatient setting, and hospital admittance in order to receive chemotherapy is rare.

After sitting in a comfortable chair, an IV will be inserted into your arm or, if you have one, your **mediport** (see Question 83). Depending on which drug you are receiving and your previous experiences with the drug, you may then be given a series of medications to help prevent side effects like nausea, vomiting, diarrhea, or allergic reactions. Following this, your chemotherapy will be administered. This may take up to few hours, depending on which drug or drugs you are receiving, as certain drugs may need to be given slowly.

Mediport

A device that is inserted underneath the skin of the chest wall that delivers chemotherapy.

The experience should comfortable and painless. If you feel any burning in your arm, you need to tell the nurse immediately as it may be sign that the chemotherapy drug is leaking into your skin. You can watch TV, read a book, work on your computer, or relax, and then eat after any nausea has subsided. Following that day's chemotherapy, you may need further IV fluid hydration. At the end of the session, you are disconnected from the IV line and can go home. You should discuss with your medical team whether or not you can drive yourself home after your treatment, as it is often not permitted if you have received medications that can make you drowsy.

Gary Rosen's comment:

This probably sounds a bit odd, but I look forward to my treatments. Everyone working at the treatment center is there to help, and the chemo nurses are some of the nicest people I've ever met. They understand what we're dealing with and have dedicated their careers to helping us and making us comfortable during the procedures.

54. What are some of the general side effects of chemotherapy?

While chemotherapy kills rapidly dividing cancer cells, it can also harm normal cells in the body that also divide rapidly, such as hair follicles, blood cells, and the lining of the intestines. These effects are known as toxicity, and can produce unwanted side effects. However, these are usually reversible, as normal cells have an inherent ability to repair and replace the destroyed cells—something cancer cells, which lack repair mechanisms, cannot usually do.

Some general side effects are expected with many chemotherapy drugs, while others are specific to a certain

You should discuss with your medical team whether or not you can drive yourself home after your treatment, as it is often not permitted if you have received medications that can make you drowsy.

drug or combination of drugs. An expected general side effect of chemotherapy is the destruction of red blood cells that carry oxygen (causing fatigue and/or anemia), white blood cells that fight infections (increasing the risk of infections), and platelets that are responsible for clotting blood (leading to bruising or, rarely, bleeding). Your physician will be monitoring these carefully through routine blood work.

Infections are easier to develop with a reduced white blood cell count, and any sign of fever should prompt a call to the physician and even a possible visit to the hospital.

While fatigue may be explained by a lower number of red cells, not all fatigue symptoms are due to low red blood cells. Patients with biliary cancers may be tired due to their illness, and the chemotherapy itself will often aggravate their fatigue. Infections are easier to develop with a reduced white blood cell count, and any sign of fever should prompt a call to the physician and even a possible visit to the hospital. Your physician may elect to give a skin injection to boost the number of white cells and reduce the infection risk. However, even with a low white cell count, this may not be possible depending on your treatment plan, level of well being, and how you have done with other treatments.

55. I am worried I may get nauseous or vomit. How are these symptoms prevented or treated?

Many chemotherapy agents cause nausea and even vomiting, but to varying extents. Because these symptoms are predictable, patients will be taught about the potential nausea and will be given supportive medications to prevent or alleviate these symptoms. Recently, very effective anti-nausea medicines have become readily available. Sometimes the nausea is only anticipatory, as just thinking about the treatment or walking in the door of the building may make a patient nauseated. This can be treated with anti-nausea medication, which is taken at home before going to your treatment or even the night before your treatment. For most patients, it is possible to completely prevent vomiting and minimize nausea.

Most importantly, it is very difficult to know in advance how you may react to chemotherapy. Patients may have no side effects, all of them, or some of them. Your medical team will provide a plan for managing and preempting nausea to you while they teach you about your treatment. Note that this plan may require you to take anti-nausea medication for several days following each chemotherapy session.

For most patients, it is possible to completely prevent vomiting and minimize nausea.

56. The combination of gemcitabine and cisplatin is a standard treatment for biliary cancers. How does this treatment plan work?

Gemcitabine (Gemzar®) and cisplatin (Paraplatin®) are two types of chemotherapy that have been proven to be an effective treatment for biliary cancers based on the results of a randomized Phase III clinical trial (see Question 65). Thus, a combination of gemcitabine and cisplatin doublet is typically the first treatment to be tried in patients with biliary cancer.

In the Phase III clinical trial mentioned above, a combination of gemcitabine and cisplatin was compared to gemcitabine alone. The clinical trial showed that patients who received the combination of gemcitabine and cisplatin generally lived longer and had better control of their disease compared to those who received gemcitabine only. It is important to note that neither therapy cures the cancer. The aim of the treatment is to control the cancer and prevent it from spreading further. This means increasing your lifespan while having the cancer, also known as **improved survival**. In certain situations your doctor may prescribe only gemcitabine for specific reasons, including limited body functions, which may prevent you from tolerating cisplatin well. Your doctor may also substitute cisplatin with another drug called oxaliplatin for similar reasons.

Improved survival

The increase of one's lifespan while living with cancer.

57. What is gemcitabine?

Gemcitabine is a chemotherapy drug used for many cancers that can kill cancer cells by causing changes to their DNA. Gemcitabine is administered through an IV infusion that typically takes around 30 minutes, though, in rare instances, your doctors may prescribe it to run over longer period of time. While it has several potential side effects, it is generally not as debilitating as other forms of chemotherapy (see Question 58). For biliary cancers, it is standard practice to infuse the gemcitabine and cisplatin together as a doublet (see Question 56), though it is common to switch to gemcitabine alone after continuing this therapy for a long while.

58. What are the side effects of gemcitabine?

You may experience one or more of the following side effects of gemcitabine, or you may experience none of them. The potential side effects of gemcitabine include, but are not limited to, a decrease in the number of your red blood cells (a condition called anemia), a decrease in your white blood cell count, and a decrease in your platelet count. A low white blood cell count increases the risk of getting an infection. While you may not require any specific extra precautions, you should wash your hands often and avoid direct contact with people with infections, colds, or flu. A low platelet count may make you prone to bruising and, rarely, bleeding.

You may have an upset stomach, feel nauseous, and even vomit. It is very likely that your doctor will prescribe anti-nausea medicine. Make sure to take your medications as advised.

Gemcitabine can cause flu-like symptoms. These include headache, weakness, fever, shakes, aches, pains, sweating, and a feeling of malaise. Loose stools or diarrhea may also occur. Your hair may thin and you may experience hair loss. However, your hair will recover upon stopping the medication. You may feel tired or fatigued. You may also notice some swelling in the feet or arms. Mouth irritation or sores can also occur.

Your hair may thin and you may experience hair loss. However, your hair will recover upon stopping the medication.

Rare side effects include damage to the kidneys and liver or the development of an inflammation in the lungs that can cause severe shortness of breath.

59. What is cisplatin?

Cisplatin, like gemcitabine (see Question 57), is a chemotherapy drug that can kill cancer cells by causing changes to the DNA of cancer cells. Cisplatin is used for many cancers, including biliary cancers.

Cisplatin is administered through an intravenous infusion. While the infusion may not take long, it can require longer chemotherapy sessions if your doctor wishes to infuse extra fluids to help flush the cisplatin through your kidneys. This is done to protect them from damage (see Question 60).

There are variants of cisplatin that your doctor may use. The two most commonly used alternatives are carboplatin and oxaliplatin. In biliary cancers, oxaliplatin is generally preferred over carboplatin. Oxaliplatin is commonly used interchangeably with cisplatin for a variety of reasons, such as protecting you from specific side effects or for schedule convenience. Your medical team will discuss such alternate choices if they are deemed appropriate.

60. What are the side effects of cisplatin?

You may experience one or more of the following side effects of cisplatin, or you may experience none at all. The potential side effects of cisplatin include, but are not limited to, a decrease in your red blood cell count (a condition called anemia), a decrease in your white blood cell count, and a decrease in your platelet count. A decreased white blood cell count can increase the risk of getting an infection. While you may not require any specific extra precautions, you should wash your hands often and avoid direct contact with people with infections, colds, or flu. You may feel tired or fatigued. You may have an upset stomach, feel nauseous, or even vomit. It is very likely that your doctor will prescribe anti-nausea medicine. Make sure you take your medications as advised. Your hair may thin or fall out, but should regrow when you stop taking the medication. You may also experience loose stools or diarrhea. Prolonged exposure to cisplatin can lead to hearing loss, and your doctor may recommend that you take regular hearing tests. You may also develop tingling in the fingers and toes (**neuropathy**), which, if not reported and followed carefully, can become permanent and may affect your abilities to do tasks like button a shirt or type at a computer.

Neuropathy

A tingling in the fingers and toes that can result from certain chemotherapy drugs.

Your doctor will follow these symptoms very closely and will reduce or stop the cisplatin if you begin to exhibit any of these symptoms. You can also develop kidney damage during your treatment. To help prevent this, your doctor may ask you to collect urine for 24 hours to obtain an accurate assessment of your kidney function, and may repeat the test on regular basis. Some patients can develop an "allergy" or "hypersensitivity" reaction to cisplatin when it is being administered as a result of being repeatedly exposed to the drug. If this reaction occurs, you may be given medication before the infusion of cisplatin to prevent the allergy and you will likely be given the cisplatin more slowly and monitored closely. Sometimes, the nature of these allergic reactions is serious enough that a decision will be made not to administer them again.

61. How will I know that my treatment is working?

You will take chemotherapy for as long as your doctor finds it helpful in fighting your biliary cancer. Your doctor may recommend stopping your chemotherapy if you are unable to tolerate it well or if it is not helping your cancer. Your doctor will rely on different factors to determine if you are benefiting from the treatment, the primary one being your general clinical condition. Questions like "Do you have symptoms?" "Did they

Your doctor may recommend stopping your chemotherapy if you are unable to tolerate it well or if it is not helping your cancer.

worsen or improve?" "Did new symptoms develop?" all provide helpful information. Doctors will routinely use a CT scan, an MRI, or an ultrasound to get an idea of how far the cancer has progressed before starting any treatment.

Your doctor may also check the levels of tumor markers in your blood, also known as cancer markers, to determine any progress. There are three types of tumor markers that are mostly associated with biliary cancers, carcinoembryonic antigen (CEA), CA 19-9, and AFP. However, these markers have not been validated as a medium to gauge the response of biliary cancers to chemotherapy. Thus, as enticing and easy as they are to follow (i.e., the fact that markers are reported as numbers, and that an increase in their total is bad while a decrease is good) the information they provide is not necessarily true. You doctor is more likely to depend on a combination of all of the signs and tests when deciding if the treatment you are currently receiving is benefiting you.

Gary Rosen's comment:

I received cisplatin and gemcitabine for 2 years. In my case, it helped shrink the tumor from 9 cm to 4 cm. The drugs took a bit of a toll on my kidneys and left my feet a bit numb, so we switched to a different combination of drugs. Yes, there are side effects, but I try not to focus on them and carry on with my life. It's been a while since there has been any shrinkage of the tumor, but, as Dr. Abou-Alfa says after my CT scans, the tumor is "stable," and stable is a good thing.

62. What kind of scan is best to assess tumor response?

Since many patients who receive chemotherapy have metastatic cancer, a CT scan or an MRI is usually used to assess the status of the cancer. Before undergoing a CT scan, you will be given an oral contrast agent to be drunk immediately before the scan. An intravenous contrast agent will also be infused into your vein. The oral contrast agent will help the radiologist assess the intestinal tract, while the IV contrast agent will help visualize tumors in your liver, blood vessels, and other areas of the body. When you undergo a CT scan, you will lie down on a table and a donut-like part of the scanning machine will circle around you, taking pictures of the interior of your body. Depending on which parts of the body are scanned, the procedure may take anywhere from 10–30 minutes.

If you undergo an MRI, you will be given an intravenous contrast agent before lying on a table that is enclosed within the scanner. You may feel uncomfortable in such a tight place. MRIs can be noisy and typically take longer than a CT scan, often lasting around 45 minutes. Talk to your doctor and/or radiologist about which is the best test for you.

Occasionally, a PET scan may be recommended after a CT scan or MRI. A PET scan involves the injection of glucose into your vein and may help determine whether a finding on a CT scan or MRI is in fact cancerous or not. You can expect to have a repeat evaluation, preferably using the same type of scan, every 2 to 4 months. The radiologist can evaluate the cancer by measuring it and looking for changes compared to the previous scan. These measurements are compared with the original

You can expect to have a repeat evaluation, preferably using the same type of scan, every 2 to 4 months. The radiologist can evaluate the cancer by measuring it and looking for changes compared to the previous scan.

CT scan or an MRI that was taken before the start of therapy and any scans taken since. The best possible result is a complete response to therapy, in which the cancer disappears completely in the radiologic scans performed. However, this is an uncommon result. Much more common is a partial response or a slight reduction in the size of the tumor.

Stabilizing the disease is another possibility and is considered a satisfactory result that can justify and support continuing the same treatment. For technical reasons, the category of stable disease is applied to a result showing 30% shrinkage of the tumor up to a 20% increase its in size, accommodating for the technical limitations and other factors using radiologic tests. It is important to factor in these considerations in when you review your CT scan or MRI with your medical team. Typically, a significant increase in the size or the appearance of new tumors represents **progression of disease**. This may be a reason to stop the current treatment and to consider a different therapy.

Progression of disease

A growth of cancer that is represented by an increase of the size or number of tumors.

63. What are tumor markers?

As part of diagnosing and following your biliary cancer, your doctor may order blood tests to detect cancer activity. These tests are often called "cancer numbers" by patients. There are three types of markers of interest in biliary cancers: CEA and CA19-9 (both of which apply to all types of biliary cancers), and AFP (which may be associated with cholangiocarcinoma). By themselves, these markers are not significant enough to tell you and your doctor how well a treatment is working, and you should never formulate an idea on how your cancer is reacting based on the numbers going up or down. It is important to note that not all cancers express these markers and if they do, they not necessarily imply that the cancer is growing or shrinking. For example, a shrinking cancer in response to treatment may secrete one or more of these markers or vice versa. Thus, these tumor markers have to be interpreted in perspective together with your general condition and the results shown in the CT scans or MRIs when trying to get a complete picture of the progress against your cancer condition. It is also important to know that tumor marker levels can significantly increase with an infection in the bile duct or with inflammation in your pancreas, conditions that may not be directly related to how your cancer is behaving.

It is also important to know that tumor marker levels can significantly increase with an infection in the bile duct or with inflammation in your pancreas, conditions that may not be directly related to how your cancer is behaving.

64. If I stop treatment with gemcitabine and cisplatin, what should I do next?

In the case that your doctor finds that gemcitabine and cisplatin are not working for you, or if you cannot tolerate this therapy, you may be offered alternative treatment options. These may include joining a clinical trial, trying out other forms of biological therapy or chemotherapy, or trying a combination of these. As there is no clearly defined optimal treatment choice if gemcitabine and cisplatin do not work out, you should inquire about whether clinical trials are suitable for you. If your medical condition has become worse, your doctor may not offer further therapy, as you may not be able to tolerate it and it may do you more harm than good. If this is the case, you may be offered palliative care.

Gary Rosen's comment:

When we stopped the cisplatin and gemcitabine treatments, I was put on two other drugs. One is systemic and the other is delivered directly to the blood supply of my liver via an intrahepatic infusion pump (see Question 69). This is an engineering marvel. It is implanted under the skin of my abdomen and it delivers a small dose of the chemo directly into the artery supplying blood to my liver. It's a small dose, but 100% of it is delivered to the target.

65. What is a clinical trial?

A clinical trial is a research study that follows and monitors the effects of a new drug or combination of drugs on a certain group of patients. Patients in clinical trials are overseen with precision. Medical researchers are working on new discoveries and treatments every day, and newly discovered therapies must be tested on patients in order to determine their safety and effectiveness.

Clinical trials can answer many scientific and medical questions. They can be used to test a single new drug or new combination of drugs, test different methods of delivering different drugs, and test new therapies. The same basic regulations generally apply to all clinical trials; however, here they are discussed here in the context of biliary cancers.

All clinical trials are, and should always be, clearly described and outlined in a document called a protocol.

All clinical trials are, and should always be, clearly described and outlined in a document called a protocol. A protocol is the primary guide to a clinical trial, as it describes all of the regulations and conditions that govern the trial. Close adherence to the protocol ensures the quality of the trial, guaranteeing its reproducibility and keeping the patients within the trial safe.

Unfortunately, there have been poorly conducted trials in the past that have exploited patients for the sake of answering a scientific question. However, this is a thing of the past, as all trials are now governed by federal regulations that protect patients. Clinical trials are also monitored by an independent committee, also called an institutional review board (IRB), which enforces the trial's protocol and any ethical considerations very strictly.

Ultimately, patients who are given the option to join a clinical trial make the decision about whether or not to participate for themselves. If a patient does enter a trial, he or she has the right to withdraw from the trial at any time. These rights, as well the details of the study, should be discussed between the patient and the medical team in a process called informed consent. This process is essential and protects the rights of all patients. If a patient elects to proceed with a study, they will typically be required to sign a confirmation that the medical team has discussed an informed consent document that outlines the objectives and details of the clinical trial. A copy of this document is provided to the patient as a permanent record.

If a patient does enter a trial, he or she has the right to withdraw from the trial at any time.

Clinical trials generally occur in several phases: Phase I, II, and, III. The primary goal of a Phase I study is to establish the safety of a newly discovered drug or combination of drugs while also getting a very early sense of the efficacy. Phase I studies are often conducted with patients with a variety of different cancers and after the standard therapies for their disease have proven ineffective. A Phase II trial studies the effectiveness of a drug or a combination of drugs in a specific type of cancer. However, the treatments efficacy is ultimately determined through a Phase III study that compares the experimental drug or drugs to the standard treatment for the cancer in question (i.e., gemcitabine and cisplatin for biliary cancers). In a Phase III trial, patients will be randomly assigned to either half of the study (experimental or standard) to ensure the validity of the experiment.

Not all patients are candidates for clinical trials. Clinical trials are designed to answer specific questions within the boundaries of specific criteria that a certain patient may not have. This does not imply that patients who are not eligible for a clinical trial should not be treated after the standard treatment has failed.

Gary Rosen's comment:

As a result of my genetic testing, I may be a candidate for a clinical trial that Dr. O'Reilly is conducting for patients with cancer and BRCA 2. This may be an option if the current therapies are no longer effective and is just another reason to consider genetic testing.

66. Where can I learn about clinical trials for biliary cancers, and how do I know which trial is best for me?

Patients should ask their medical team about clinical trials. Many doctors, both at academic centers and in private offices in the community, run or are part of a group of doctors running a clinical trial, meaning the answer could be right at the patient's doorstep. Nonetheless, patients might consider commuting a distance to a center that runs a pertinent clinical trial for their cancer. Patients can learn about these trials through either their medical team, the cancer center's website, or either of the National Cancer Institute (NCI) websites: *www.cancer.gov* or *www.clinicaltrials.gov*. The NCI offers not only a listing of all clinical trials, but also several web pages with information about clinical trials. Other sites that offer similar services include the Coalition of Cancer Cooperative Groups, *www.cancertrialshelp.org*, and CenterWatch, *www.centerwatch.com*. Additionally, patient advocacy organizations often have information relating to clinical trials.

If a patient identifies a clinical trial that is relevant to his or her medical condition, he or she should discuss the trial further with his or her medical team. If a patient is deemed ineligible for a certain trial, he or she should not be. It is important to know that certain clinical trials answer only a specific question in a specific subset of patients with a given disease. For example, a new drug for biliary cancers may be tested in only patients who have a specific type of biliary cancer, such as intrahepatic cholangiocarcinoma.

It is important to know that certain clinical trials answer only a specific question in a specific subset of patients with a given disease.

67. What are biological therapies? Are there any specific new biological drugs being tested for biliary cancers?

Recently, scientists have achieved a better understanding of how cancer cells grow and evolve, including the specific steps in cell reproduction that lead to uncontrolled replication of cells, causing cancer. They also have identified specific therapies that can stop tumor replication or disrupt a tumor's blood supply. These new therapies and their targets, also known as a targeted therapy, operate like a key and a lock. While some therapies, or keys, are specific to certain cancers, or locks, others may have an effect on many different targets, like a master key. As with other cancers, these new "targeted" or "biological" therapies may play a role in treating primary biliary cancers. Although doctors call these drugs "targeted therapies," they are not as precise as one might think and can have side effects similar to chemotherapy.

Unlike other cancers, no definite biological therapy has proven effective for biliary cancers so far. However, many are currently under study, including classes of drugs that interfere with blood vessel growth and development (anti-angiogenic drugs) and drugs that interfere with various signaling pathways that are important in cancer cells. If you were to be offered participation in a clinical trial, it is very likely that it will include at least one of these biological drugs.

68. What is cancer genetic sequencing?

In an attempt to find out which target may be part of your cancer and thus allow your medical team to prescribe the most appropriate medication, researchers have recently begun to genetically sequence, or profile, different cancers, biliary cancers included. The process consists of determining the precise order of the basic elements, called nucleotides, within the DNA of your cancer. By identifying unique genetic changes associated with your cancer that differ from normal cell DNA, your medical team is able to prescribe a currently available targeted therapy or refer you to a clinical trial that is looking at a drug for a specific target.

Biliary cancers involve many genetic changes, so it is difficult to pinpoint one or two specific targets.

The problem, especially in biliary cancers, is that scientists are not yet sure of what to look for or which targets are relevant. Biliary cancers involve many genetic changes, so it is difficult to pinpoint one or two specific targets. Because of this, you may get a wealth of information about your cancer that may be currently unusable by your medical team. However, the good news is that this field is evolving very rapidly, so it is always good to discuss these options with your medical team. Genetic sequencing is available and may or may not be covered by your insurance company. Genetic sequencing is also part of many clinical trials aimed at helping doctors around the world better understand the genetic makeup of both biliary cancers and cancer in general. While the information learned during the trial may or may not benefit you directly, you may be helping future fellow cancer patients.

69. What is liver pump chemotherapy?

Some patients might have biliary cancer that is either confined to or has spread only to the liver. In some circumstances, the tumor can be very large, can involve major blood vessels, and is not operable, or there can be multiple tumors scattered throughout the liver. These circumstances would not be suitable for surgery, transplant, or any other of the local therapies previously discussed. However, there may be an option to send chemotherapy drugs directly where they are needed in the liver, thus maximizing their effectiveness against the cancer and minimizing any possible side effects to other parts of the body. This type of chemotherapy, called liver-directed or **hepatic artery infusion (HAI)** chemotherapy, entails having a catheter inserted into an artery that leads to your liver, through which chemotherapy drugs are infused.

Typically, this placement requires an operation to place the pump and catheter, and requires a special liver CT scan before the surgery to determine if your blood vessel anatomy is suitable for this type of approach. A

Hepatic artery infusion (HAI)

Chemotherapy that is delivered directly into the liver via a catheter in the hepatic artery. This is ideal for cancers that are confined to the liver.

Typically, if HAI chemo-therapy is being given, it is given along with IV chemotherapy in order to maximize drug delivery to the liver in addition to reaching all parts of the body.

surgically inserted HAI pump can be accessed from the outside with a needle through the skin. The pump acts as a reservoir and slowly releases the drugs into the liver over a 2-week period of time. The main drug used in this type of chemotherapy is called floxuridine (FUDR), which is a version of the drug 5-fluorouracil, an IV drug commonly used in the treatment of many abdominal cancers, including biliary cancers. HAI chemotherapy is not a proven approach, although data from clinical trials has indicated that is useful form of treatment for some patients with biliary cancers where the cancer is not operable. It is also being studied as a preventative approach after complete removal of the cancer. Typically, if HAI chemotherapy is being given, it is given along with IV chemotherapy in order to maximize drug delivery to the liver in addition to reaching all parts of the body.

Gary Rosen's comments:

As previously indicated, I have a liver pump. It is about the size of a small hockey puck and is implanted under the skin of my abdomen. They change the drug every 2 weeks, switching between chemo and saline. There is no battery, as it is driven by the heat of my body. It's an innovative way to introduce the drug, as it feeds directly into the blood supply of my liver. This means that 100% of the drug is delivered to the target. One note regarding the pump: sky diving, scuba diving, and going into hot tubs are no longer permitted, as they can have an effect on the pump's flow. Oh well.

70. What is radiation therapy?

Radiation therapy uses the high energy of electromagnetic waves to kill cancer cells. These powerful radiation rays can be controlled and directed toward cancer cells, killing them. The two main types of radiation waves used in radiation therapy are X-rays and gamma rays. They differ in production and power, and have different applicability in cancer treatment.

Currently, there are two main forms of radiation therapy. One, known as external beam radiation, usually consists of X-rays and is delivered from outside of the body, penetrating the skin and targeting where the tumor resides. The second form of radiation, called **brachytherapy**, uses gamma rays that are produced radioactive material inserted or implanted inside the body near the tumor.

New radiation techniques are constantly being developed and vetted in an effort to maximally focus the radiation on the tumor and to minimize the effects on the surrounding normal cells. These new techniques include giving higher doses of radiation for a shorter period of time, and may require special procedures to set up the radiation, including the placement of fiducials or "markers" into the tumor to help direct the radiation. You may also be instructed to use certain breathing techniques during the delivery of the radiation to ensure the radiation hits only where needed and that it would not be affected by your breathing movements.

71. Can radiation be used for the treatment of biliary cancers?

Although radiation is a commonly used form of treatment for many cancers, its role in general biliary cancers is somewhat limited by the liver's reduced ability to tolerate radiation. Generally, the radiation will be applied to the liver no more than 10 times. These are typically delivered 5 days a week over a 1–2 week period. In the

TREATMENT

Brachytherapy
A radiation treatment method that delivers radiation therapy inside the body directly to a tumor. This is done through a radiation therapy implant that can be placed during surgery.

New radiation techniques are constantly being developed and vetted in an effort to maximally focus the radiation on the tumor and to minimize the effects on the surrounding normal cells.

past, such treatments typically radiated the entire liver and could cause inflammation, as part of a condition known as **radiation hepatitis**.

Radiation hepatitis

Liver inflammation as a result of radiation treatment.

Today, radiation hepatitis can be avoided by using localized radiation therapy to radiate only the cancerous parts of the liver. Radiation oncologists) can prepare a three-dimensional computer model of the liver and the tumor. This helps them to target the radiation, which is then emitted in small amounts from many different sources toward a very localized portion of the tumor. Together, all of these small emissions will cause damage to the tumor while keeping impact on the surrounding liver tissue to a minimum.

Radiation therapy can be combined with chemotherapy and used to treat locally advanced, inoperable biliary cancers. Additionally, newer techniques like **intraoperative radiotherapy (IORT)**, which applies radiation directly to the bile ducts, and **intensity-modulated radiation therapy (IMRT)** represent a technical advance in dosage delivery and the minimization of toxicity.

Intraoperative radiotherapy (IORT)

A form of radiation treatment that delivers radiation directly to the bile ducts.

Intensity-modulated radiation therapy (IMRT)

A form of radiation therapy that helps deliver a high amount of radiation to the cancer while avoiding surrounding normal tissues.

The tendency for cholangiocarcinoma to recur locally provides a rationale for additional local adjuvant or preventative therapy after definitive surgery (see Question 42). However, the indications for postoperative radiation therapy are not clear and there is no consensus on which patients should be recommended for radiation. It is recommended that you discuss the benefits and risks of treating your cholangiocarcinoma this way with your medical team. There may also be clinical trials for adjuvant chemotherapy and radiation available to you, so be sure to check with your doctor or on *www.clinicaltrials.gov.*

72. Are there other uses for radiation?

Radiation can be used to help relieve pain at sites where the cancer has spread to the bones. It also may be used preventively to avoid a bone fracture at any weak, weight-bearing sites (e.g., the hips) the cancer has spread to. Additionally, radiation can be used to reduce the size of cancer sites in the vertebrae in order to prevent them from compressing the spinal cord, causing pain and even paralysis. Spinal cord compression is an emergency condition that requires prompt medical attention. If at any time you develop any arm or leg weakness (especially a weakness on one side), have a decreased sensation in any of the extremities, or if you lose control of urine or stools, you need to call your doctor immediately, as these may be signs of spinal cord compression. This condition is typically treated by either surgery or radiation. Steroids can also be given to help reduce any inflammation that may contribute to the symptoms.

73. What are complementary and alternative treatments? How do I decide whether I should use one of the complementary or alternative therapies that my family or friends are recommending?

Complementary and alternative medicines include acupuncture, homeopathy, and naturopathy among others. Many cancer centers around the country now have integrative medicine departments or sections that offer alternative therapies to patients. These include, but are not limited to, alternative medical acupuncture, homeopathy, and naturopathy. Diet and nutritional advice are other components. For the mind and body, many facilities offer psychotherapy, meditation, hypnosis, biofeedback, and massage, among many others. These may also include herbal remedies.

While a great deal of research has identified some of these therapies as effective, many have yet to be studied in depth. Discuss your interest in these approaches with your doctor, who will refer you to an integrative medicine doctor. Avoid taking any medicines on your own before discussing them with your medical team. Remember that many of today's medicines may be composed of components similar to those that comprise the alternative ones that you may be considering, which can result in overdosing. By the same token, many of the medicines that are labeled as natural or herbal can have potential adverse effects and can interact negatively with your treatment. Do not hesitate to discuss alternative therapies with your medical team. Bring any pills and/or herbs that you are interested in with you, and always try to have a list of the ingredients. This might help your doctor to identify any potentially beneficial or harmful products.

Avoid taking any medicines on your own before discussing them with your medical team.

Gary Rosen's comment:

Most folks think of vitamin and mineral supplements as good and don't realize that they can interfere with treatment. Vitamin C is considered by many to be somewhat harmless. However, I found some research by a doctor at MSKCC indicating that large doses of vitamin C, taken before treatment with cisplatin, can reduce the effectiveness of the chemo drug. I take no supplements unless I am instructed to by my oncologist.

74. What if my doctor recommends that no treatment should be performed?

Some patients are not eligible for any of the previously discussed treatments. Your doctor may decide that it is too risky to treat you if your cancer is too advanced, if your body is too weak, or if you have other significant medical problems. In this situation, your doctor will offer the best supportive care possible. You should not perceive this approach as though your doctor or you are "giving up." Avoiding treatment may protect you against things that could get worse if you were to be treated. This means that your medical team will try to help with any symptoms that develop and try to maximize your quality and length of life. This is called palliative care. You may not necessarily experience any pain, but if you do, pain medications can and should be prescribed. Some patients also may require assistance living at home, and often a social worker or case manager can help arrange for a healthcare professional to visit you at home.

You may not necessarily experience any pain, but if you do, pain medications can and should be prescribed.

75. How should I use the Internet to learn about my cancer? What about social media?

The Internet is a vast resource for medical information. You may learn about a specialty center near you or discover a clinical trial in which you can participate. Although many doctors recommend that you learn about your cancer, they will warn you that you may find information that is not relevant to your individual situation,

TREATMENT

Through social media websites, you may be able to communicate with other patients who have your cancer, which may help you cope with the problems that you are facing.

which can lead to confusion or fear. Thus, although it is valuable for you and your family to learn about biliary cancers, you should discuss your Internet research with your doctor. Remember that some websites are more reputable than others. Look at who runs the website and learn whether there is any supporting staff you can contact with questions. Be sure that your confidentiality as a patient is kept while navigating such sources on the Internet. Through social media websites, you may be able to communicate with other patients who have your cancer, which may help you cope with the problems that you are facing. However, you must be cautious about certain websites, as many are not monitored and any data or information you see needs to be placed in context.

Gary Rosen's comment:

I initially did a lot of searching on the Internet for information on cholangiocarcinoma. I soon realized that it is a difficult subject and that it was depressing. I've stopped these searches, other than an occasional look at clinical trials. When I have questions, I ask my doctor when I am in the clinic or via the secure patient portal.

PART SIX

Cancer-Related Practical Issues

I feel overwhelmed by all of the information that I am receiving. How do I make any decisions regarding my treatment?

Will changing my diet affect my cancer?

I feel tired. What can I do to help with fatigue?

More...

76. I feel overwhelmed by all of the information that I am receiving. How do I make any decisions regarding my treatment?

The amount of information you will receive following your diagnosis can feel overwhelming. This sentiment is understandable and even expected. While it's good to know of all your options, it can be daunting. Take notes, but do not immerse yourself in details so that you are able to keep the big picture in mind.

In many cancer centers, you may be taken care of by a medical team. Your medical team will consist of a group of physicians who will all be talking to each other, and who will be discussing decisions regarding your cancer and working closely with one another. Typically, one physician will be in charge, though who it is depends on the phase of your illness and your therapy. For example, your surgeon will usually be in charge if your main therapy is operation, while your medical oncologist will often take the lead if you are receiving chemotherapy.

77. Will changing my diet affect my cancer?

Omitting sugar, while a popular remedy on the Internet, has not been proven to help eradicate cancer.

This is a common question among patients with cancer. In general, no specific diet recommendations exist for cancer patients, though most doctors will encourage you to eat a balanced diet and begin taking a multivitamin.

Proteins are always encouraged to maintain and increase muscle mass. Omitting sugar, while a popular remedy on the Internet, has not been proven to help cure or treat cancer. If you are on chemotherapy, it is recommended that you avoid raw meat and fish, as your white blood cell count may drop. Also, be sure that your unpeeled fruits and vegetables are thoroughly washed.

Gary Rosen's comment:

For the record, I have not eaten meat, pork, or poultry for over 40 years. I have followed a modified vegetarian diet since 1970, but still developed cancer. I recommend that you follow your doctor's advice and not fall for any "quick fix" or fad diets.

78. I am concerned I am losing weight. Can I do something about it?

Weight loss is a common problem for people with biliary cancer. Having cancer changes your metabolism, which results in your body needing many more calories each day than are consumed in a normal diet. In addition, symptoms of the cancer or side effects from the treatment may make it difficult to consume enough nutrients and fluids. You may have no desire for food (**anorexia**) or feel full after only a few bites of food (early satiety). You may find that food tastes different or that symptoms such as nausea, gas, or constipation make it difficult to eat. Pain, fatigue, or emotional distress can also affect your appetite. In addition, changes in how your body digests or absorbs food may make it difficult for your body to use the nutrients and fluids you do take in.

Anorexia

A side effect of cancer or its treatment that causes a person to lose his/her appetite.

Consuming enough food and fluids is important to providing energy to your body and in helping you to handle treatment.

Consuming enough food and fluids is important to providing energy to your body and in helping you to handle treatment. For these reasons, maintaining your normal weight or reducing the amount of weight that you are losing, if possible, are important. You can do a number of things to improve your appetite and to help maintain your weight.

Medication may be helpful if you are having symptoms (e.g., mouth sores, nausea, vomiting, diarrhea, constipation, pain, or emotional distress) that affect your appetite. Ask your doctor for medication to relieve these symptoms. Also, following certain types of biliary surgery, especially surgery for extrahepatic bile duct cancer, many people do not secrete enough digestive enzymes for food to be digested and absorbed. This may cause changes in your stool, gas, and loss of weight. If you feel that this is happening to you, ask your doctor about taking pancreatic enzymes by mouth. In addition, there is a medication called megesterol acetate (Megace®) that may improve your appetite. Other medications that are considered in certain circumstances include mirtazapine (Remeron®), dronabinol (Marinol®), or olanzapine (Zyprexa®). Ask your doctor if any of these medications could help you.

It is also helpful to make changes in your diet to maximize the amount of nutrients that you take in each day:

- Eat small amounts of food and fluids at a time. Rather than trying to eat three full meals a day, eat six or eight snacks throughout the day. Always have food nearby to nibble on.

- Select foods high in protein and calories. Foods rich in these that many people find easy to eat when they are not very hungry include eggs, cottage cheese, yogurt, peanut butter on crackers, sandwiches with turkey or tuna fish, baked or broiled chicken, fish, or beef, and soups.

- Add a variety of ingredients to recipes to enhance the flavor of food and add calories (e.g., butter, honey, jelly, sour cream, cheese, yogurt, cream, and evaporated milk). *Eating Hints for Cancer Patients*, published by the National Cancer Institute, provides many helpful recipes. More eating tips can be found at *www.cancer.gov/cancertopics/coping/eatinghints/page1.*

- Experiment with different foods and different seasonings to find those that taste the best to you. Some people find that red meat does not taste as flavorful while getting chemotherapy; chicken and fish may taste better.

- Limit the amount of fluids that you drink with your meals so that you don't fill up on the fluid.

- Limit the amount of caffeinated beverages (e.g., coffee, tea, and many sodas) that you drink, as these will cause dehydration.

- Limit the amount of carbonated beverages that you drink, as they will make you feel full.

- Replace fluids with no nutritional benefit (such as water or soda) with fluids that provide nutrients (such as cream soups, shakes, and fruit smoothies).

- Try nutritional supplements that are available in your local drugstore. These may be canned drinks, powders to be mixed with water or milk, or puddings. Your doctor or nurse may recommend specific supplements for you. You can also use Carnation Instant Breakfast by blending it with milk and adding ice cream, yogurt, and/or fruit.

You may also want to rinse your mouth with water before eating, as moistening your mouth may enhance the taste of your food. Try not to eat alone. Having company can make eating more enjoyable, and we often eat more when eating with someone else.

It is common for family members and friends to recommend special diets, high-protein drinks, or supplemental megavitamins and antioxidants. Like anything suggested by outside sources, these should not be taken without first speaking with your medical team, as they may interfere with your treatment, be dangerous, or detract from your nutrition.

Family members who have worked hard to prepare special foods may feel frustrated if you push it away after only a few bites. Avoid conflicts, but remind them that you are only able to eat what your appetite allows. Remember that eating should be pleasurable. The most important thing is to eat what you want when you want it, though you should always try to keep your nutrition in mind. In some cases, you may find it helpful to speak with a registered dietitian (certified by the American Dietetic Association) for guidance about what to eat. If so, ask your doctor or nurse for a referral to a nutritionist with expertise in working with people who have cancer.

Remember that eating should be pleasurable. The most important thing is to eat what you want when you want it, though you should always try to keep your nutrition in mind.

Gary Rosen's comment:

My weight tends to go up and down. Upon receiving my diagnosis, I stopped worrying about limiting my diet, thinking the end was near. Now, I try to control myself, but do allow myself some treats on occasion. I have experienced very little nausea over the past 4.5 years, but my biggest challenge from the treatments is regulating my bowels. Try to be conscious of your bowel movements, but don't obsess over it. I find that a few dried apricots help when things aren't moving regularly.

79. I feel tired. What can I do to help with fatigue?

Fatigue is a common symptom for patients with cancer and can be attributed to many factors. The cancer itself, especially in its advanced stages, may tire people. In addition, chemotherapy can cause fatigue, which may require an adjustment of the dose of the drug or drugs you are being given. Some chemotherapy drugs can cause a drop in the number of your red and white blood cells, which also can contribute to fatigue. If this leads to anemia, your doctor may recommend red blood cell-transfusion or treat you with iron supplementation. Up until several years ago, doctors prescribed an injection that could boost your red blood cell count. Now, this injection is only given in rare instances, as recent data has emerged that links the injected red blood stimulation agents with increased mortality, serious heart problems, and cancer progression. If these agents are recommended, you should have a thorough discussion with your medical team regarding the risks and benefits.

Mental fatigue is another symptom. It can result from travel, your many medical appointments, ongoing tests, and the concerns and fears that come with being diagnosed with cancer. You can avoid mental fatigue by focusing on daily goals and keeping notes on events so that you do not burden yourself trying to keep track of too much information. Keep it simple, and remember to always look at the big picture.

Remember that it is okay not to think about your cancer all of the time. You need to energize and be ready for the next step and taking a break from "the cancer" can be very helpful.

Many relatives, friends, and colleagues will be calling to check on you. It is very good to have people around, and your doctors will always encourage you to maintain your social support group. Remember that it is okay not to think about your cancer all of the time. You need to energize and be ready for the next step and taking a break from "the cancer" can be very helpful.

Pain may be another cause of fatigue. Ensuring that your pain is well controlled is an important part of medical care.

80. I am experiencing pain. How can I stop it?

Pain needs to be controlled, as it may affect your mood and your level of daily functioning, and it can cause you to become more ill and tired. You need to tell your medical team about pain, as it can be alleviated. Mild pain usually responds well to acetaminophen (Tylenol®) or nonsteroidal anti-inflammatory drugs (NSAIDs) such as Motrin® and Advil®. Acetaminophen should be taken with caution, however, as taking excessive amounts of it can affect liver function. Make sure that you tell your doctor how much acetaminophen you are taking so that they can assess its safety. Be careful with NSAID medications as well, as they can cause bleeding or kidney damage.

If these medications are not enough to control your pain, you may be prescribed opiate-based medications called narcotics. Many variations of these medications exist, and they are divided into two main categories: short-acting and long-acting. If your pain is limited, then your doctor most likely will prescribe a short-acting narcotic such as morphine or oxycodone to be taken in doses of one to two pills several times a day. These may be sufficient for controlling your pain. Examples of the short-acting opiates include a combination of Tylenol and oxycodone, such as Percocet®. Your doctor may avoid prescribing these medications if there is a risk of liver damage due to too much acetaminophen. If you require many short-acting pills to control the pain, your doctor may elect to add a long-acting narcotic taken twice a day in pill form, such as Oxycontin® or MS Contin®, or as a skin patch (Fentanyl®) that is applied every 3 days. Although the patch appears to be easier, you still may be prescribed pills due to allergic concerns, personal preference, or poor absorption caused by reduced body fat.

The aim is for the pain to be minimized or, ideally, eliminated. Remember that your pain medication requirements may increase over time due to a natural phenomenon called tolerance (this should not be mistaken with addiction). Your pain can also get worse, leading to you requiring more medication to control it. You are strongly encouraged to speak about your fears and concerns with your medical team. Sometimes specialist pain management physicians may be involved in your care if you have had troublesome side effects from the pain medication or your pain has been difficult to control.

The aim is for the pain to be minimized or, ideally, eliminated.

Like all medications, opiates have side effects. You may feel sleepy or drowsy, especially when you first begin taking them. This usually dissipates after a few days. If it persists, your medications may need to be fine tuned to reach a comfortable level in terms of both pain control and side effects. However, you should never operate any machinery or drive while taking opiates. If you require high doses of pain medication, you may sleep

You may have more or less side effects with different types of opiates. Sometimes, switching to different medications may help ease some of the side effects.

for long periods of time. While your family and friends may want to see you awake and speak with you, controlling your pain should be more important. Constipation is another side effect. You may become constipated while on opiates, and you will likely need to maintain a daily regimen of a stool softener such as Colace® and a laxative such as Senekot®, Miralax®, magnesium citrate, or Lactulose®. Drinking fluids will also help keep your bowels functioning regularly.

You may have more or less side effects with different types of opiates. Sometimes, switching to different medications may help ease some of the side effects.

81. How do I prevent or relieve nausea and/or vomiting?

Nausea and vomiting have long been considered to be unavoidable side effects of cancer treatment; however, with the recent development of new anti-nausea medications (antiemetics), this is no longer the case. Both radiation therapy to the abdominal area and chemotherapy may cause nausea or vomiting. This can result from irritation of the stomach or from chemical stimulation of areas in the brain that trigger nausea and vomiting. Vomiting is when you throw up stomach contents through your mouth. Retching, gagging, or dry heaving all feel similar to vomiting, but cause no stomach contents come up.

Whether or not you develop nausea or vomiting depends on many things, including which chemotherapy drugs you are receiving. The most commonly used chemotherapy drugs for treating biliary cancers (gemcitabine and cisplatin) cause nausea or vomiting in most patients if they receive no anti-nausea medication. Approximately 50% of people undergoing radiation therapy to the abdominal area experience nausea or vomiting if they receive no anti-nausea medication. With medication, the likelihood that you will experience nausea or vomiting with either treatment is much lower.

People vary widely in their reactions to the same treatment: Some have very severe nausea, some have more mild nausea, and still others experience no nausea or vomiting at all. For people who do experience nausea or vomiting, the timing of these symptoms will also vary. Some patients develop symptoms within minutes or hours after treatment, while others develop symptoms days later. The symptoms may last several hours for some and many days for others. Some patients experience their most severe symptoms before leaving home for or while on their way to treatment; this is called anticipatory nausea or vomiting.

Many effective ways of managing nausea and vomiting are available, but the most important is the use of medication. These medications are most commonly given orally, intravenously, or by inserting a suppository into the rectum. Taking your treatment and the timing and severity of your symptoms into account, your doctor will prescribe a specific anti-nausea medication for you. You may be instructed to take the medication at home either before going to or after returning from your treatment, or the nurse may give you medication immediately before your chemotherapy. Different anti-nausea medications work in different ways, and if one medication is not effective, you should call your doctor or nurse and ask for a different medication.

Different anti-nausea medications work in different ways, and if one medication is not effective, you should call your doctor or nurse and ask for a different medication.

Medicine is not the only method of controlling nausea, however. Techniques that use your body and mind, such as guided imagery, self-hypnosis, and progressive muscle relaxation, can be very helpful, particularly with anticipatory nausea or vomiting. Ask your doctor or nurse for a referral to someone trained in these techniques if you are interested in learning one of them. Also, some people find it helpful to minimize the use of things in the home that have particularly strong odors (e.g., perfumes or certain cleaning products).

Changes in what you eat and drink may also help to manage nausea and vomiting. Some specific suggestions include the following:

- Eat a light meal before each treatment.
- Consume food and fluids in small amounts.
- Consume bland foods and fluids, avoiding spicy foods and foods with strong odors.
- Eat dry crackers when feeling nauseated.
- Limit the amount of fluids that you take with your meals.
- Drink enough between meals, taking in clear fluids such as water, apple juice, herbal tea, or bullion. Additionally, some people find that carbonated sodas are helpful, while others find flat soda to be better.
- Eat foods at or just below room temperature.
- Avoid high-fat, greasy, and fried foods.
- Avoid alcohol and caffeine.

Taking in enough fluids and nutrients is important for your health. If you are unable to keep any food or fluids down for 12 hours or if you are only able to take in small amounts of food or fluids for 24 hours, call your doctor or nurse.

82. I cannot sleep at night. What can I do to sleep better and feel more rested?

Difficulty falling asleep in the evening or staying asleep throughout the night are common problems for people with biliary cancer. Aside from the distress caused by lying awake in bed, not getting enough sleep may cause you to have trouble concentrating and to feel irritable and tired throughout the day.

First, try to determine the cause of your sleeplessness. Are you physically uncomfortable or in pain? Are you having other symptoms (e.g., nausea, vomiting, diarrhea, constipation, itching, mouth sores) that are making it difficult to sleep? To get a restful night's sleep, it is very important to take medication as prescribed to treat these problems. If you are taking medication and it is not effective, tell your doctor or nurse.

Are you feeling anxious and worried during the night? Are your thoughts racing and keeping you awake at night? Speaking with someone whom you trust and feel supported by about your thoughts and feelings may provide a significant amount of relief. For some people, taking anxiety medication may be helpful.

If you are suffering from more of a general restlessness at night and are unable to relax and sleep, there are a variety of techniques that can be helpful:

- Establish a regular time to go to bed each night.
- Even if you do not sleep well at night, try not to sleep too much during the day. This will disrupt your body's normal cycle. If you are very tired, take only a short nap during the day (about 1 hour).

- Avoid being in bed at any time except when you are going to sleep. When resting during the day, lay in another room on a couch or chair. Use your bed only for sleep at night.
- Avoid drinking caffeine or other stimulants after dinner.
- Try a method of relaxation.

For some people, however, these techniques are still not helpful. If you continue to have difficulty sleeping, ask your doctor to prescribe a sleeping medication. Getting a restful sleep will help you to feel energized and capable during the day.

Gary Rosen's comments:

On the evening following my treatment, I find it difficult to get a good night of sleep as a result of the steroids. Since I have to go to work the next morning, I take a sleeping aid. On other days, I sometimes wake up in the middle of the night. To distract my thoughts, I turn on the TV, set the timer, and watch something light. Generally, I fall asleep quickly and don't see more than a few minutes of the program.

83. What is a mediport?

A mediport is a device that can be used to deliver chemotherapy. It may be necessary if the patient has limited intravenous access in their arms or if the chemotherapy is to be delivered while the patient is at home. A mediport is inserted underneath the skin of your chest wall by a surgeon or an interventional radiologist. The procedure takes about 45 minutes and is performed while you are lightly sedated.

A mediport has two components: a reservoir and a catheter. Both are inserted beneath the skin on your chest close to your shoulder. The reservoir is about the width of a half dollar and may be visible as a small lump just below your collarbone. When beginning a chemotherapy session, a nurse will insert a needle connected to an IV through your skin into the reservoir. The drug, or any other intravenous solution, then passes through the reservoir, down the catheter, and into your body.

There are several complications that can stem from a having a mediport, including a 1% chance of having one of your lungs collapse while the device is first being inserted. If this does occur, a small tube will be inserted into your chest to remove the excess air that can collapse the lung if left alone. A much more common complication is infection. Because a mediport is a foreign object in your body, there is a chance that it may lead to an infection-caused bacteria infecting the mediport. The risk of an infection can be decreased by having only experienced persons in a sterile environment access it. Blood clots are another more common complication. Because the catheter attached to the reservoir sits in a vein, this vein may develop a clot. Your doctor may request that you take start on a blood thinner while you have a mediport, as this can help prevent a clot from forming. If either an infection or a blood clot occurs, your mediport may need to be removed.

Because a mediport is a foreign object in your body, there is a chance that it may lead to an infection-caused bacteria infecting the mediport.

Gary Rosen's comment:

For me, the mediport was a tremendous help. After almost 2 years of treatments, it became a challenge for the chemo nurses to find a good vein in my arms. Since the mediport was put in, I no longer have pain or difficulty from blood tests or treatments. I understand that sometimes it is not indicated, but, if your doctor recommends it, get one.

PART SEVEN

Biliary Cancer–Specific Issues

I have been told I have jaundice.
Why are my eyes and/or skin yellow?

How is a mechanical bile duct blockage fixed?

More...

84. I have been told I have jaundice. Why are my eyes and/or skin yellow?

Jaundice is a condition caused by accumulation of bile in the body, often as a complication of liver failure. However, in patients suffering from a biliary cancer, jaundice is more likely to be caused by a blockage in the bile ducts due to the cancer. The tumor may press on a bile duct and not allow the bile to drain the normal way into your gallbladder and intestine and instead backs up in the liver, causing jaundice. Your doctors may recommend a stent (a type of plastic or metal pipe) to overcome the blockage or a diverting procedure in order to decrease the build-up of bile and so that you can be treated with chemotherapy. This may also relieve you of symptoms like severe itching.

By itself, jaundice is not dangerous, and, at worst, it can cause itching that can be treated with a medicine like Benadryl®. However, the presence of jaundice may prevent you from having surgery or receiving therapy for fear of further damaging your liver.

Gary Rosen's comment:

Before the stent was put in, I became quite jaundiced. I was still working and I would sit in my office with the door closed and the lights out. I was uncomfortable and very self-conscious, and I avoided speaking with my coworkers. The stent brought relief and has worked well. I continue to go into the office, with the door open and the lights on.

85. What is the difference between a stent and a drain?

If the blockage is accessible, you will have a plastic or metal stent inserted in order to open a collapsed bile duct. Sometimes this it is not possible because of the location of the blockage or other technical reasons. If this is the case, a catheter may need to be inserted through the skin and into the liver to drain the bile to the outside of your body through an opening in the side of your abdomen. This catheter is open on both ends: to the outside through the skin and through your liver to your intestines. Outside of your body, the catheter is hooked to a plastic bag that can be secured under your clothes below the insertion site at your waist or around your leg. Bile collects into the bag that must be emptied and changed periodically, either on your own or with the help of a nurse.

A stent is always preferred over a catheter, as it is a closed system that is not exposed to the outside, which decreases the risk of infection. A catheter can be replaced with a stent after some time, allowing the bile to drain into your intestine. This avoids having the drain stick out of your body for convenience and safety purposes. This can usually be done when the bile pressure goes down, which is indicated by bile no longer coming through the catheter and into the bag. If this occurs, your doctor may test to see if the catheter can be "internalized" and converted to a stent. Your doctor will "cap" the external drain and monitor it for a few days, looking for worsening jaundice, abdominal pains, or fever, any of which imply that the catheter is not working inside of your body. If this occurs, you will likely be required to use the catheter for a longer or even indefinite amount of time.

A stent is always preferred over a catheter, as it is a closed system that is not exposed to the outside, which decreases the risk of infection. A catheter can be replaced with a stent after some time.

BILIARY CANCER-SPECIFIC ISSUES

86. *How is a mechanical bile duct blockage fixed?*

A "mechanical blockage" refers to the duct being blocked by the actual tumor. A stent can be inserted to relieve this type of blockage through either an endoscopy or through an incision made into the side of your abdomen, while a catheter requires an incision to be inserted. If it is being inserted through an endoscopy, a gastroenterologist will conduct the procedure after you have been lightly sedated. During an endoscopy, a scope is piped through your mouth down into your intestine. The stent is then fed through the scope into the bile duct opening in your intestine.

If the stent is being inserted through an incision or if you require a catheter, the procedure will be carried out by a team of interventional radiologists. You will first be lightly sedated, and then a small incision will be made in your abdomen. Through this the stent or catheter will be fed into your bile duct, with the radiologists using X-ray imaging to guide their work

Both of these procedures will likely require you to not eat after midnight the night before the procedure. If there is a concern about infection, the procedures may have to be performed emergently. Following either procedure, you are likely to be admitted to the hospital and observed for a few days. It may take several days for your bile level level to drop low enough for you to start your cancer treatment again.

87. *What are the risks associated with a biliary catheter and how do I care for it?*

One of the main concerns with stents and catheters is infection. It is important to note that your bile ducts are normally sterile, meaning that no bacteria grow within them. Once a stent or catheter has been inserted, however, your bile ducts become colonized with bacteria from both the intestine and from outside your body, as your bile ducts now are open to the outside and are exposed to bacteria. These bacteria can cause an infection at anytime, especially if you have been fitted with a catheter, as the drain provides a constantly open system to the outside. Because of this, it is imperative to keep your biliary catheter and bag as clean as possible and to follow the exact instructions you are given on how to take care of them. If an infection occurs, your catheter will be opened if it has already been closed with a cap and you will likely be admitted to the hospital and started on intravenous antibiotics. There is the possibility that you will be able to go home and finish the antibiotic regimen in pill form. In the case of some infections, you may need to stay on prophylactic or preventative antibiotics indefinitely to prevent further infection. Complications of an infection include bleeding and damage to the bile duct, and can require hospital admittance. These complications are rare and are more likely to occur at the time of the insertion of the stent or drain.

While stents and catheters can be a very valuable part of your care, they can also be a source of serious complications that you may want to avoid altogether. In general, your doctor, in collaboration with your interventional radiologist or gastroenterologist, should be able to give you a sense of how successful an intervention of this kind will be. If the likelihood of success is low because of difficulty to reach a blockage or because of the potential need for several catheters, you and your doctor may decide to forgo this approach and resort to palliative care (see Question 93).

88. My abdomen and/or legs are swollen. What is edema? What is ascites?

Proteins help our blood vessels retain fluids, and in their absence, fluids start seeping out of the blood vessels into are called "third spaces."

If your biliary cancer becomes worse, your nutrition can become very poor. This is often because your body cannot keep up with your protein demands, as a substantial part of the protein you ingest is consumed by the cancer itself. Proteins help our blood vessels retain fluids, and in their absence, fluids start seeping out of the blood vessels into are called "third spaces." These are typically the legs (peripheral **edema**), abdomen (ascites), and groin areas of the body.

Edema

The collection of fluid in parts of the body.

The lack of protein may also be due to poor liver function and the development of cirrhosis. Blood pressure can build up inside the liver, causing what is called portal hypertension. This causes the body to start accumulating more water and salt, which ultimately leads to swelling in the abdomen or in the legs.

A third possible cause of fluid build-up in your abdomen is the direct spread of the cancer to the lining of the abdominal wall, which is also known as the peritoneum. This can also cause inflammation and the build-up of water, which can be quite substantial and may result in bloating, feeling full, swelling of the abdomen, pain, weight gain, and shortness of breath.

89. How do you treat edema and ascites? What is a paracentesis?

Many factors contribute to edema and ascites (fluid in the abdomen), including, poor nutrition, cirrhosis (liver malfunction), and spread of the cancer to the peritoneum. Unfortunately, there is little that can be done to eradicate these factors, but this does not mean nothing will be done to help manage your symptoms. Your doctor will typically try to slow the accumulation of fluids, potentially through several different methods. The simplest way may be to restrict salt intake, as salt draws water with it. You might even need to restrict your salt intake to less than 2 grams of salt (800 mg of sodium) per day; for reference, one slice of bread has about 500 mg of salt. Your doctor also may prescribe a diuretic such as spironolactone (Aldactone®), or a combination of diuretics by adding furosemide (Lasix®). These actions are typically effective in keeping the fluid retention at a steady level. However, your doctor may need to drain the fluid or ascites from your abdomen by using a catheter. This procedure is called a paracentesis and is a straightforward, bedside procedure that can be done with or without the help of an ultrasound to locate the fluid. During the procedure, you lie on your back, possibly turning more toward your right. Your doctor will sterilize one spot of your skin, usually in the left lower corner of your abdomen. You will be administered a shot containing a weak local anesthetic to numb the area. Afterward, your doctor will insert a needle with a catheter that will drain the clear, yellowish fluid into a bottle or a bag. Your doctor will judge how much fluid should be removed to make sure that your blood pressure and other vital signs are not affected by this rapid change of body fluid. The procedure carries a small risk of infection or bleeding and can also lead to the loss of proteins.

The management of ascites and edema can be a very challenging task. In situations where the fluid reaccumulates rapidly, your medical team may recommend placing a semi-permanent catheter called a Tenckoff or PleurX catheter into your abdominal cavity. These types of catheters are inserted by an interventional radiologist while you are under light sedation and are left in place. You and/or your caregivers will be taught how to drain the fluid once to twice daily to reduce reaccumulation. The major risk of having this type of catheter in place is the risk of an infection in the abdominal wall (cellulitis) or infection of the inner lining of the abdominal cavity (peritonitis).

PART EIGHT

Family, Social, and End-of-Life Issues

I feel depressed. How can I get help?

Can I work during treatment?

What if my doctors suggest stopping my current therapy?

More...

90. I feel depressed? How can I get help?

As detailed in Question 25, depression is common among patients with cancer and can present different symptoms. You may feel sad, have difficulty concentrating or remembering details, and find it hard to make decisions. You may feel tired, have trouble sleeping at night, and sleep more during the day. You may also feel irritable and restless, and find yourself less interested in the activities or hobbies you once enjoyed. You may not feel like eating. If the depression condition is advanced, you may also start to feel anxious, guilty, worthless, or even suicidal. If you find you are having these types of thoughts, you should speak with your doctors or loved ones about them immediately. Handling depression may help you better combat the cancer both physically and mentally. Your doctor may refer you to a psychiatrist. If you have signs of depression, it is highly advisable that you follow this recommendation. A psychiatrist may start you on medications to combat your depressive symptoms, anxiety, and lethargy. Your psychiatrist may not call your condition depression but rather an adjustment disorder, which refers to your difficulty adjusting to a major stressor like cancer.

Handling depression may help you better combat the cancer both physically and mentally.

91. Can I work during treatment?

Most patients with biliary cancer are able to return to work after recovering from surgery. Patients undergoing chemotherapy are typically able to continue working during their treatment, but can require longer periods of rest following each session, and so may only be able to work part time. If your condition and energy level allow for it, you should continue to work, as it will help maintain a sense of normalcy in your life.

If your condition and energy level allow for it, you should continue to work, as it will help maintain a sense of normalcy in your life.

Make sure to discuss your thoughts and concerns with your doctor. If you are currently employed, you are most likely entitled to sick days or an unpaid leave. You can check the U.S. Department of Labor Medical Leave Act of 1993 at *www.dol.gov/whd/fmla/index.htm* to learn more. You also may need to review your disability benefits. The benefits department at your place of employment should be able to discuss all of the benefits to which you are entitled.

You may be nervous or unsure about telling your supervisor or coworkers about your cancer diagnosis, and it is up to you to decide how much, if anything, you wish to share. It is important to remember that you should not fear being treated differently or discriminated against. The Americans with Disabilities Act protects you against discrimination at work and also requires your employer to make reasonable accommodations for you as long as you are able to perform the essential functions of your job. You may need to discuss your work schedule, limitations, and other aspects of your job with the company's human resources department. If any conflicts arise from you asserting your rights, you may wish to contact a lawyer. Additionally, you can contact the U.S. Department of Justice at 800-514-0301 or at *www.usdoj.gov/crt/ada/adahom1.htm*.

It is important to remember that you should not fear being treated differently or discriminated against.

Remember that your supervisor and coworkers may feel uncomfortable learning of your diagnosis, either due to previous family experience or out of fear of a disease that they do not know much about. For those who are interested, try to educate them; for those who decide to alienate you, remain kind and courteous. With time, as they watch you continuing to function like any other person, their fears and anxieties may dissipate and your relationship may go back to what it was.

Gary Rosen's comment:

With all of the stuff I've had to deal with relating to my condition, I consider myself very fortunate. I work in New York City, and the firm I work at is a few blocks from the treatment center. My bosses have been incredibly supportive. On treatment days, I work for a few hours, walk across town, get my treatment, and take the train home. I don't always feel 100% after a treatment, but keeping my daily routine helps me cope. Working each day keeps me from focusing on my condition. It gets me out of the house, gives me some exercise when I walk in the city, and allows me to speak with different folks. My cancer is always there, but it doesn't consume my thoughts throughout the day.

92. What if my doctors suggest stopping my current therapy?

If the cancer becomes too advanced and resistant to therapy, or if your body becomes too weak to tolerate any treatment, your doctor may elect to stop all active therapies. While this may cause you to feel angry, upset, or helpless, it is important to remember that they are not giving up on you. Rather, your doctor is actually trying to protect you from any harm that your treatment could cause and instead concentrate on alleviating any symptoms that you have, focusing on palliative care (see Question 93).

93. What is palliative care?

Palliative care
Active care that is concentrated on symptom management.

Palliative care is care that is concentrated on treating and controlling symptoms. It is an active approach and you will still see your doctor regularly. Topics you can expect to discuss include your symptoms, such as jaundice, as well as your pain control, nutrition, and any other concerns that you might have. Controlling your symptoms at this stage of your cancer will allow you to maintain some functionality in your life. You should use this time to do things like visit your family and friends, travel to your favorite places, enjoy your hobbies, or attend religious services. Keeping a positive and hopeful attitude is the key to remaining content and peaceful through this period of time.

Keeping a positive and hopeful attitude is the key to success at this stage.

94. What is hospice?

If your medical condition worsens, you may become debilitated and need a great deal of help and support. This can be provided through hospice care. **Hospice** is a whole-system care approach that addresses medical, physical, emotional, social, and spiritual needs for patients with advanced-stage disease. This care can be provided at home, especially if your family is able and ready to provide the physical care. A hospice registered nurse and possibly a hospice care physician will visit you on a regular basis and as frequently as is necessary. These regular assessments will ensure that you remain comfortable and that all of your needs are addressed. The hospice care team will consult regularly with your doctor. If necessary, you may be provided with a home health aide to assist you with your physical needs, such as bathing. Although the hospice caring team will be present at your home for only a few hours a day, these resources are available 24 hours a day, 7 days a week in case an emergency arises.

Hospice
Care approach that addresses many different needs (medical, physical, emotional, social, spiritual) for patients with advanced disease. Hospice care can be provided in the patient's home or at a hospice facility as an inpatient.

You also may have hospice care provided at a hospice facility as an inpatient. This can be because of personal wishes, the nonavailability of family members, or if you require strenuous care that your family members cannot provide. You can still have quality time with your family and loved ones at an inpatient hospice facility, as most have extended visiting hours. Meanwhile, the staff will provide all of the care that you need.

You are entitled to hospice care after you and your doctor decide not to pursue any further active care, such as chemotherapy, and your doctor may recommend hospice care if your cancer is life threatening. Additional information is available at *www.hospice-info.net* and *www.hospicenet.org*. Some hospice facilities provide palliative care or specific spiritual care. You can discuss with your doctor what options are available or visit the website of the National Hospice and Palliative Care Organization at *www.nhpco.org*.

95. What are advanced directives?

Considering the advanced nature of your cancer, you may want to provide your medical team with advanced directives regarding your end-of-life care. Advanced directives are legal documents that are made to protect your wishes for end-of-life care and to ensure that they are carried out. The two basic forms of advanced directives are a living will and a healthcare proxy (see Question 96)

In a living will, you may state specific instructions that relate to your medical care in case you are unable to communicate them.

In a living will, you may state specific instructions that relate to your medical care in case you are unable to communicate them. It should state clearly your wishes if your heart stops beating or you stop breathing, two events that can occur in the advanced stages of cancer. Your doctor may offer a short version of a living will that addresses those two issues. Treatments that you may request in the event of your heart stopping include cardiopulmonary resuscitation (CPR), defibrillation, or the infusion of medications to speed up your heart. The failure of your lungs can be treated by connecting them to a breathing machine via intubation, a process in which a tube is inserted down the trachea. This is called being on life support.

While these interventions can resuscitate you, it is important to take into account both your comfort and the terminality of your condition. For patients with very advanced cancers, these treatments may seem tormenting, painful, and nondignifying and are very unlikely to succeed in reviving you. As such, your doctor may recommend that you give a do-not-resuscitate (DNR)/do-not-intubate (DNI) order in your living will. Have an open and frank discussion with your doctor about DNR/DNI orders to make sure that you understand them fully. Discuss those wishes in advance and do not leave them until it is too late. When you are comfortable and do not feel pressured, you are better able to make a rational decision. Remember that a DNR/DNI order does not limit your access to medical care in any way and issuing one will not impact the treatment course that you already on.

Your living will also might include wishes that relate to drawing blood, giving blood, feeding, dialysis, and the like. Make sure that all of this is discussed fully with your doctor. Generally, your doctor will not recommend any invasive measures unless they will truly improve your chances of survival. Otherwise, your doctor will guide you to make a decision that would improve your comfort. Remember that in medicine, sometimes doing less is doing more.

Gary Rosen's comment:

I have a living will and DNR/DNI on file at MSKCC. It's difficult enough for my wife and daughters, and I don't want them to have any doubt how I would want to be treated if I am no longer able to communicate. I feel that I owe it to them to address these issues.

96. What is a healthcare proxy?

The second part of an advanced directive is the assigning of a healthcare proxy. A healthcare proxy is someone you have appointed to make healthcare decisions on your behalf if you are not able to because of your illness. This is very important, as some states do not recognize living wills, and, even if they do, some decisions not previously discussed with you may need to be made while you are asleep, unconscious, or simply unable to make them. In those instances, your healthcare proxy (also called a health surrogate, a medical proxy, or a medical power of attorney) will act on your behalf and make those decisions.

A healthcare proxy should be a friend or family member whom you trust to make decisions based on your wishes, both stated and unstated. Before assigning one, make sure to inform whomever you have in mind of your interest in assigning them as your proxy.

A healthcare proxy should be a friend or family member whom you trust to make decisions based on your wishes, both stated and unstated. Before assigning one, make sure to inform whomever you have in mind of your interest in assigning them as your proxy. Make sure that they are comfortable with that decision. If they are, be sure to have a candid and honest discussion about your wishes to ensure that they both know and are comfortable with them. In order to avoid any unnecessary conflicts, it is important that you inform your friends and family of who is your healthcare proxy. You can discuss healthcare proxy issues with your care team, social worker, patient representative, or lawyer.

Gary Rosen's comments:

My wife and daughters have been established as my proxy. They know my feelings and will make the decisions if I cannot. This is important, because you don't want the state or some stranger making decisions about your treatments.

97. What should I do to prepare to die? Where can I find hope?

Although the concept of death can be frightening, preparing for it might help erase that fear and cast it as more of a transitional phase that is an integral part of our life cycle. Thinking about death does not mean you are giving up but rather are gaining an opportunity to help you shape the end of your life. The earlier that you begin preparing the better, as you do not want to feel pressured or disappointed if things do not go the way you wish.

Clearing up your financial issues is one of the first things you should do. Work with your attorney, accountant, and your family in order to do so. You may need to write a will, especially if you have family members who are financially dependent on you. Sort out your financial plan and keep your attorney's name and contacts available. Also, keep all legal, financial, and health documents organized for easier access.

Additionally, remember to visit with your loved ones, family, friends, and colleagues. Get in touch with loved ones who live far away. If you are troubled by any unresolved issues you have with someone, work on sorting them out. Indicate to whom you want to give any valuable items you have. Photographs you possess are memories that celebrate your life and can be passed from one

Thinking about death does not mean you are giving up but rather are gaining an opportunity to help you shape the end of your life.

119

generation to another. You may wish to prepare some aspects of your funeral. This is a celebration of your life and an important closure for everybody.

For many, the biggest fear is leaving loved ones, especially children, behind. To help with this, be sure to see them as often as you can. Preparing a photo album or scrapbook about your lives together can help, as can starting or continuing to write in a diary. In doing so, you are creating artifacts through which you can be remembered and celebrated.

If you are ever feeling overwhelmed or hopeless, try to recall and imagine your dearest moments. You will notice that you are full of life.

As you can imagine, you may be quite busy regardless of how close death is. If you are ever feeling overwhelmed or hopeless, try to recall and imagine your dearest moments. You will notice that you are full of life.

98. Where can I find additional information?

Throughout the book, many resources have been referenced that can help you to get additional information or answers to your questions. In this era, the Internet can be a great resource that pertains to many aspects of your biliary cancer.

On many websites, this information is periodically updated, so it can be quite accurate. However, it is still important to be cautious when taking and using information found on the Internet, as some sites may have information that is not verified or that is out of date. Always check with your healthcare team if you are in doubt. Online chat rooms or forums can be another resource that helps you to share your experience and exchange information with others. If you wish to participate in any of these discussions, it is important to remember that no two patients are alike, so any information or advice given to you in either of these settings should be evaluated with a critical eye before you act on it. A comprehensive cancer center can provide you with additional resources available as well. Always make sure to ask because you will be amazed at how much care and support are available.

99. How can I help other patients?

Many patients find it gratifying to reach out to others with the same cancer and offer them support and guidance based on their experience. You may be able to offer support explaining the processes involved in doctor's visit, the diagnosis, and the management of your biliary cancer. Such interactions can take place through a one-on-one agreement that may be facilitated by your physician's office, with the help of your medical team and the agreement of you and the other patient, or through support groups that are established locally or nationally.

100. Are there foundations who help/support biliary cancers?

The Cholangiocarcinoma Foundation (*www.cholangiocarcinoma.org*), the American Liver Foundation (*www.liverfoundation.org*), and the Foundation for Awareness of Gallbladder & Bile Duct Cancer (*www.gallbladdercancersurvivor.com*) are just some of the non-profit foundations that provide help, advocacy, and educational resources for patients, families, and caregivers.

Gary Rosen's comment:

Cholangiocarcinoma is quite rare, and it's to our advantage to support these organizations. As indicated, they provide visibility to these disorders and drive research for conditions that could easily be ignored.

A

Ablation: The destruction of tissue internally, without removing it. Examples include alcohol injection, cryotherapy, irreversible electroporation, and hepatic artery embolization.

Abscess: The development of an infection in dead tissue.

Adenocarcinoma: Type of cancer that develops in organs that have a tube structure, like the colon, or bile ducts. It is also called glandular cancer.

Adjuvant therapy: Treatment given after surgery to lessen the chance of the cancer's recurrence.

Anemia: A condition marked by a lowering of the red blood cell count, resulting in fatigue.

Anorexia: A side effect of cancer or its treatment that causes a person to lose his/her appetite.

Ascites: A condition in which the abdomen is distended with fluid.

B

Bile: A liquid secreted by the liver that helps in the digestion of food, particularly fatty foods.

Bile ducts: Thin tubes in the liver that carry bile.

Biliary cancer: Cancer of the bile ducts.

Biliary tree: The collection of all the bile ducts.

Biological therapy: A type of therapy that operates like a key against a specific cancer target or a lock. While some therapies, or keys, are specific to certain cancers, or locks, others may have an effect on many different targets, like a master key.

Body surface area: A measurement of size based on a person's height and weight.

Brachytherapy: A radiation treatment method that delivers radiation therapy inside the body directly to a tumor. This is done through a radiation therapy implant that can be placed during surgery.

C

Cadaveric transplant: An organ for transplantation taken from a person who is brain-dead, but whose organs are still alive.

Cancer: The growth and division of cells in an unregulated fashion, which impedes the normal cell cycle.

Cancer staging: A system of measurement that describes the extent of the cancer, measuring tumor type (T), involvement of lymph nodes (N), and whether the cancer has metastasized (M).

Caroli disease: A condition, also known as choledochal cysts, in which bile ducts dilate and make cyst-like structures; can be a risk factor for cholangiocarcinoma.

Cell cycle: The control of cells by orderly signals that indicate when they should grow and divide.

Chemoembolization: A treatment plan that uses both chemotherapy and hepatic artery embolization.

Chemotherapy: The use of medication to kill or stop the growth of cancerous cells.

Cholangiocarcinoma: Cancer that originates in the major bile ducts in the liver.

Cholangiography: A technique involving puncturing the skin and passing a small tube through the liver and into the bile ducts under X-ray guidance.

Cholangitis: Infection involving symptoms such as fever, shaking chills, severe abdominal pain, and worsening jaundice. This infection is sometimes caused after bacteria are introduced into the bile duct system after an ERCP or percutaneous intervention to relieve jaundice.

Choledochal cysts: A condition in which bile ducts dilate and make cyst-like structures; can be a risk factor for

cholangiocarcinoma. Also known as Caroli disease.

Cirrhosis: A liver disease, often a result of alcoholism or hepatitis that can complicate the treatment of biliary cancers.

Cisplatin: A chemotherapy drug that causes cell death by changing the DNA of the cancer cells.

Clinical trial: A research study that seeks to test new treatment options for a disease.

Common bile duct: A duct that is formed by the joining of the common hepatic duct and the cystic duct. The common bile duct travels through the pancreas and opens into the duodenum.

Colonoscopy: Endoscopic examination of the bowel with a camera on a flexible tube passed through the anus. It can be used for visual diagnosis and biopsies.

Common hepatic duct: The main duct of the liver through which bile ducts exit.

Computed tomography (CT) scan: An X-ray that produces images of sections of the body.

Cryotherapy: A procedure involving the insertion of a metal probe into tissue and freezing it, thereby destroying the tissue.

Cystic duct: A duct that leads from the gallbladder and joins with the common hepatic duct.

Cytotoxic drug: Medication that is used to kill or stop the growth of cells, especially cancerous cells.

D

Duodenum: The first section of the small intestine.

E

Echocardiogram: An ultrasound of the heart.

Edema: The collection of fluid in parts of the body.

Electrocardiogram: An imaging test that produces tracings of the heart.

Endoscopic retrograde cholangio-pancreatography (ERCP): A procedure in which an endoscope (camera) is inserted into the stomach through the esophagus to visualize the performance of various procedures, including placing a stent or metal tube in bile ducts to relieve jaundice.

Extrahepatic bile duct cancer: Cancer that involves the bile ducts outside the liver. These cancers are found at the joining of the liver and the extrahepatic bile ducts and are also known as Klatskin tumors.

G

Gallbladder: A small, rounded, hollow organ that stores bile and sits outside the liver in the upper right side of the abdomen. The gallbladder squirts bile into the duodenum, especially after the consumption of fatty foods.

Gallbladder cancer: Cancer that starts in the gallbladder.

Gastroenterologists: Physicians whose practice focuses on the gastrointestinal tract.

Gastritis: Stomach irritation.

Gemcitabine: A chemotherapy drug that causes cell death by changing the DNA of the cancer cells.

Genetic testing: Direct examination of a person's DNA obtained from blood, the mouth, or a tumor. Genetic testing is valuable when concerning heritable diseases and certain cancers.

H

Hematoma: A large bruise.

Hepatectomy: Removal of the liver.

Hepatic artery: The artery that supplies blood to the liver.

Hepatic artery embolization: A procedure that involves the injection of substances into the blood vessels of a tumor.

Hepatic artery infusion (HAI): Chemotherapy that is delivered directly into the liver via a catheter in the hepatic artery. This is ideal for cancers that are confined to the liver.

Hepatocellular carcinoma: Cancer that starts in the liver.

Hepatologists: Physicians who focus on the liver and its ailments.

Heptobiliary surgeons: Surgeons who specialize in operating on biliary and liver cancers.

Hospice: Care approach that addresses many different needs (medical, physical, emotional, social, spiritual) for patients with advanced disease. Hospice care can be provided in the patient's home or at a hospice facility as an inpatient.

I

Improved survival: The increase of one's lifespan while living with cancer.

Integrative medicine: A growing discipline in the medical field that addresses the medical needs, along with the emotional, social, and spiritual needs, of patients and their families.

Intensity-modulated radiation therapy (IMRT): A form of radiation therapy that helps deliver a high amount of radiation to the cancer while avoiding surrounding normal tissues.

Intrahepatic cholangiocarcinoma: Cancer that arises from the major bile ducts inside the liver.

Interventional radiologist: A physician who utilizes minimally invasive, image-guided procedures to diagnose and treat cancers.

Intraoperative radiotherapy (IORT): A form of radiation treatment that delivers radiation directly to the bile ducts.

Irreversible electroporation (IRE): A procedure that uses electricity to destroy tissue.

J

Jaundice: A condition marked by a yellowing of the skin and eyes and a darkening of the urine, possibly due to an obstruction of the bile ducts.

K

Klatskin tumor: Extrahepatic bile duct cancers that are located very close to where the bile ducts exit the liver.

L

Laparoscopy: A surgical procedure that uses a fiber-optic camera.

Liver resection: Surgery that removes part of the liver.

Living donor: A person who is still alive who chooses to donate an organ; this is typically a family member or friend of a patient.

M

Magnetic resonance cholangiopancreatography (MRCP): A specialized form of MRI performed before an ERCP that helps visualize the details of the bile duct, cancer, and obstruction.

Medicaid: Government-provided health insurance available to people who are unable to receive health insurance another way.

Medicare: Government-provided health insurance available to people over the age of 65.

Medical oncologist: A doctor whose focus is in diagnosing cancer, managing it, and treating it using methods including chemotherapy, targeted therapy, and biological therapy.

Mediport: A device that is inserted underneath the skin of the chest wall that delivers chemotherapy.

Metastasis: The process of cancer cells invading other organs directly or spreading via the blood stream and lymphatic channels to other areas of the body.

Magnetic resonance imaging (MRI): A medical imaging test that produces images of the internal organs.

Multidisciplinary care: An approach in medicine that involves a team of healthcare workers, including surgeons, medical oncologists, interventional radiologists, radiation oncologists, and other specialists specific to what's being treated.

Mutation: Change.

N

Neoadjuvant therapy: Treatment given before surgery to enhance the possibility of a successful surgery and to improve the outcome of the disease.

Neuropathy: A tingling in the fingers and toes that can result from certain chemotherapy drugs.

P

Palliative care: Active care that is concentrated on symptom management.

Pathology report: A medical report that describes important features of a disease. With cancer, it describes the type of cancer and degree of differentiation, both of which may affect the prognosis.

Patient-controlled anesthesia (PCA): Pain medication that is delivered intravenously by the patient.

Perineural: Concerning the nerves.

Positron emission tomography (PET) scan: A test that involves the injection of a sugar tracer into the body, which causes cancer cells to light up, in hopes of identifying the origin of the cancer.

Porcelain gallbladder: Calcification in the wall of the gallbladder.

Portal vein: The vein that supplies blood to the liver.

Portal vein embolization: A procedure in which a substance is injected into the portal vein on the tumor to decrease blood flow to it, stimulating the other side of the liver to grow.

Post-embolization syndrome: A condition that occurs following a hepatic artery embolization with symptoms such as fever and an increase in blood levels of liver enzymes. This syndrome usually resolves in a few days to several weeks.

Preadmission testing: Standard testing before undergoing anesthesia that involves blood tests, an electrocardiogram, and a chest X-ray.

Primary sclerosing cholangitis: A condition in which bile ducts become inflamed and blocked that can eventually lead to cholangiocarcinoma.

Progression of disease: A growth of cancer that is represented by an increase of the size or number of tumors.

Pseudoaneurysm: A weakened sidewall of a blood vessel that can break or bleed easily.

R

Radiation: A treatment that aims to kill cancer cells by using electromagnetic waves, which can be controlled and directed toward cancer cells.

Radiation hepatitis: Liver inflammation as a result of radiation treatment.

Radiation oncologist: A physician who uses ionizing radiation to treat cancer.

Radioactive bead ablation: A procedure in which small beads that contain radioactive material, known as microspheres, are injected into the blood vessels that directly feed the tumor in order to kill it.

Radiofrequency ablation (RFA): A procedure that involves the insertion of a metal probe into tissue to heat it up in order to kill the tissue.

Recurrence: The return of a cancer after it has been treated and gone into remission.

S

Sclerosing cholangitis: A condition in which bile ducts narrow, causing irregularities.

Social security: Government-provided financial assistance available to people over the age of 65 or who earn little or no income.

Social security disability: Government-provided financial assistance available to people who earn little or no income due to a disability.

Stent: A piece of plastic or metal that is used to open a collapsed opening in the body.

Systemic therapy: A type of treatment that can attack the cancer throughout the entire body, no matter where it is or it might go.

T

Targeted therapy: Medication that specifically targets the cells needed for cancer growth.

Tumor marker: A protein that is secreted into the blood. Tumor markers may be elevated in biliary cancers. Tumor markers that are important in biliary cancers include CEA, CA 19-9, and AFP.

U

Ulcerative colitis: A condition in which the gut or intestines is/are inflamed; can be a risk factor for cholangiocarcinoma.

Ultrasound: A medical imaging test that produces images of the internal organs.

Unknown primary: A cancer for which the origin is unknown.

Esophagogastroduodenoscopy (EGD): A minimally invasive diagnostic endoscopic procedure that visualizes the upper part of the gastrointestinal tract up to the duodenum.

V

Varices: Enlarged blood vessels at risk of major bleeding.

Vascular: Concerning the blood vessels.

W

Whipple procedure: A procedure that involves the removal of the lower part of the bile duct, the gallbladder, the head of the pancreas, and the duodenum, and reconnects the pancreas to the stomach and the bowel to the pancreas and stomach.

Whole body CT scan: An X-ray that produces images of larger portions of the body than a regular CT scan, covering the chest, abdomen, and pelvis.

proteins, 88
    lack of, 108
protocol, clinical trial, 74
pseudoaneurysm, 59
pulmonary emboli (PE), 47

R

radiation, 50
    for biliary cancer treatment, 81–83
radiation hepatitis, 82
radiation oncologists, 41
radiation therapy, 51, 80–81
radioactive bead ablation, 34
radiofrequency ablation (RFA), 34
    for cholangiocarcinoma, 59–60
recurrence, 36
Remeron®. *See* mirtazapine
RFA. *See* radiofrequency ablation

S

scan for assessing tumor response,
    71–72
sclerosing cholangitis, 8, 9
screening methods for biliary cancers,
    11
Senekot®, 96
sleeplessness, 99–100
social security, 31
social security disability, 31
squamous cell carcinoma, 5
staging, 21
stent, 16, 106
    and catheters, 107
    and drain, difference between, 105
stress test, 42
supportive care, 25
systemic therapy, 35, 61–62

T

targeted therapy, 32
    for biliary cancers, 77–78

Tenckoff, 110
thrombosis, 55
tolerance, 95
toxicity, 63
tumor ablation for
    cholangiocarcinoma, 56
tumor markers, 18, 72–73
    types, 70, 72
tumor, node, and metastasis (TNM)
    classification, 19
Tylenol®. *See* acetaminophen

U

ulcer, 47
ulcerative colitis, 8
ultrasound, 14, 18
United Network for Organ Sharing
    (UNOS), 53
unknown primary, 14
UNOS. *See* United Network for
    Organ Sharing
U.S. Department of Justice, 113
U.S. Department of Labor Medical
    Leave Act, 113

V

varices, 38, 47
vascular, 19
vomit, prevention of, 64–65, 96–98

W

weight loss, 89–92
Whipple procedure, 39, 45
whole body CT scan, 14

X

X-rays, 81

Z

Zyprexa®. *See* olanzapine